The

COLLABORATIVE PARTNERSHIP APPROACH TO CARE

A Delicate Balance

The

COLLABORATIVE
PARTNERSHIP
APPROACH TO CARE

A Delicate Balance

Laurie N. Gottlieb and Nancy Feeley

With Cindy Dalton

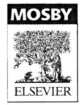

MOSBY
ELSEVIER

Library and Archives Canada Cataloguing in Publication
Gottlieb, Laurie Naomi
        The collaborative partnership approach to care: a delicate
balance/Laurie N. Gottlieb and Nancy Feeley, Cindy Dalton.
Rev. ed.

Includes bibliographical references and index.
ISBN-13: 978-0-7796-9982-7   ISBN-10: 0-7796-9982-3
        1. Nurse and patient. I. Feeley, Nancy. II. Dalton, Cindy. III. Title.
RT86.3.G68 2006 610.73'06'99 C2005-904255-9

Publisher: Ann Millar
Managing Developmental Editor: Martina van de Velde
Developmental Editor: Dawn du Quesnay
Projects Manager: Liz Radojkovic
US Publishing Services Manager: Deborah L. Vogel
US Project Managers: Katherine Hinkebein and Ann E. Rogers
Copy Editor: Lorretta Palagi
Cover, Interior Design: Paula Ruckenbrod
Typesetting and Assembly: SPI Publisher Services
Printing and Binding: Maple-Vail

Elsevier Canada
1 Goldthorne Ave., Toronto, ON, Canada M8Z 5S7
Phone: 1-866-896-3331
Fax: 1-866-359-9534

ISBN-13: 978-0-7796-9982-7
ISBN-10: 0-7796-9982-3

Transferred to digital printing 2009

To my husband, Bruce Gottlieb,
who through thought and deed embodies
the essence of collaborative partnership
—*LG*

To my husband, Wayne Kilbourne,
the true expert on collaborative partnership
—*NF*

PREFACE

The notion of a collaborative partnership between nurse and person may appear to be a new and novel form of the nurse-person relationship. It is not. The idea of collaborative partnership has been around for several decades and has long been the desired approach to working with people in the health promotion and illness prevention arenas of care (Cameron, 2004; Hartrick, 2004). We speculate that collaborative partnerships were able to take hold easily in these arenas because people feel less vulnerable, are more apt to want to partner with professionals, and have a greater voice in their own care.

The downsizing, mergers, and reorganization of the health care system of the 1990s in Canada and across the world resulted in major upheavals. Nothing escaped scrutiny. As with any form of revolution—and this has been nothing short of a revolution—old rules are being rewritten and new ones created. This has been and continues to be a time of experimentation. Even patients who are acutely ill are seeking a different role for themselves and want a different relationship with their health care provider. Collaborative partnership, once the purview of health promotion and illness prevention services, is now finding its way into more mainstream illness care services.

The authors of this text were educated at McGill University, Montreal, Canada, where collaborative partnership has been the central feature of McGill's approach to nursing. McGill School of Nursing was founded in 1920, the second university school of nursing in Canada. The first program was a post-RN diploma in public health, which might account for the emphasis on partnership with patients. Bertha Harmer, the second director of McGill School of Nursing, in her book, *Essentials of Nursing Care,* wrote about the centrality of the patient and family in care. (Later editions of this book were written by Virginia Henderson and became the primary nursing textbook for several generations of nurses.)

In the early 1970s, Dr. Moyra F. Allen, professor of nursing at McGill University, identified the core concepts of what distinguished McGill's approach to nursing from other approaches and brought these ideas together to formulate a coherent model (Allen, 1977). She originally called McGill's unique approach to nursing *situation-responsive nursing* to underscore the importance of the nurse responding to and working with the patient's needs, wants, and particular situation. Allen defined situation-responsive nursing as the nurse being responsive to the needs of people in their search for healthy family life and healthy living styles. Nursing care, therefore, was not predetermined nor decided *a priori* by the nurse alone, but was to be determined jointly by both the nurse and the person. In fact, many interpreted Allen's original conceptualization to imply that the person's goals were the only basis for determining the plan of care, and the nurse's major role was to carry out the person's wishes rather than to have input into determining the goals of care.

The idea of situation-responsive nursing has evolved and has been subsumed within a broader view of the nurse-patient relationship, which we now call *collaborative partnership*. This was one aspect of a particular perspective of nursing that is currently known as the McGill Model of Nursing. The McGill Model of Nursing provides direction to nurses as to the focus and scope of nursing care (i.e., health, development, learning, family) and how to nurse (i.e., exploratory, tailoring, strengths, collaborating). The process of nursing is collaborative; the person or family is the central focus of care, a valued partner. Nursing revolves around the joint nurse-patient agenda and goals to promote health through development: health within illness. Another aspect within the McGill Model of Nursing is the idea of learning and development. In a collaborative relationship, partners are learning from each other and learning about the health situation. In the process of learning, the person and family change and develop from this experience, as does the nurse. Every encounter with a client provides a learning opportunity and a growth experience on both a professional and a personal level.

The McGill Model of Nursing stresses the importance of working not only with the person but also with the other people who are significant influences. At the individual level, the most significant source of influence is often the family. The nurse strives to develop a collaborative relationship with an individual as well as with a family. Furthermore, the idea of developing collaborative partnerships applies to nursing with any group or collective that influences or shapes the health of individuals or a population (for example, nursing families, nursing groups, or nursing at the community level). Although the focus of this book is on individuals and families, the ideas and principles that are described are equally applicable to these populations.

Another central concept of the McGill Model of Nursing is the idea of focusing on and working with the person's strengths rather than focusing on deficits or weaknesses. *Partnership* implies that each partner brings something to the relationship and has something to contribute. Focusing on the person's strengths and working collaboratively go hand in hand. To develop a collaborative relationship with a person, the nurse begins with the expectation that the person brings to the relationship knowledge and skills (i.e., strengths) that will enable them to engage in some form of partnership. (For further information on published and unpublished papers about the McGill Model of Nursing, the reader is directed toward a compilation of writings titled *A Perspective on Health, Family, Learning, and Collaborative Nursing: A Collection of Writings on the McGill Model of Nursing* [Gottlieb & Ezer, 1997].)

This book is long overdue. There is growing interest in a collaborative partnership approach to care within nursing and among many health care professions. Although the idea of collaborative partnership has found acceptance in mainstream thinking about the relationship between health care professionals and care seekers, few have been able to actually describe how these ideas play out in practice. Perhaps this is because, to some, the idea of collaborative partnership may appear simple. It is not, however, as simple or as easy as it seems. It is a complex process requiring highly developed interpersonal and communication skills.

Although many books and thousands of articles in the nursing and behavioural sciences (psychology, sociology, anthropology, women's studies, business, and management) deal with collaborative relationships, these bodies of literature deal primarily with the nature of the relationship *between professionals* (such as multidisciplinary and interdisciplinary teams, employees and their employers) and not with the relationships between professionals and those to whom they provide service. After an extensive review of relevant databases, we located hundreds of articles that made reference to the idea of collaborative partnership between health provider and person/patient, but most failed to fully describe the nature of this partnership. Furthermore, of these hundreds of articles, only a small fraction were empirically based research studies.

Substantive literature exists on the nurse-person relationship, but little of it exclusively focuses on a collaborative type of relationship between health care professionals and the people they care for. Despite the increasing popularity of collaborative partnerships and the fact that many nursing and other scholars and practitioners advocate the adoption of this approach, we were unable to locate any book dealing exclusively with this topic. We were surprised by this, given that collaborative partnership has been our way of conceptualising the nurse-patient relationship from the inception of our nursing careers. We felt it was time for a book such as this.

Within the McGill nursing community, a critical mass of clinicians, educators, researchers, and administrators has subscribed to these ideas for more than 30 years. The ideas and principles of collaborative partnership have taken hold in different clinical practice settings with diverse populations. As a result, much has been learned about collaborative partnership in practice. *The Collaborative Partnership Approach to Care: A Delicate Balance* brings together some of the insights discovered.

In preparation for writing this book, we assembled a panel of expert clinicians, many of whom hold a joint faculty position at the McGill University School of Nursing. We held a series of group interviews to explore these expert clinicians' ideas about how to use the collaborative partnership approach in practice. (You can read more about the interviews and the experts themselves in a later section titled "Our Panel of Expert Clinicians.") One unique feature of this book is the many quotes taken from these interviews to illustrate ideas about collaboration and to help illustrate how these theoretical ideas are translated into practice. This book will help you understand what underlies collaborative partnership and will give you specific strategies that you can use to apply these ideas in your practice.

This book is written for students at all levels as well as clinicians who want to adopt a collaborative partnership approach to care. Although the main focus is on nursing, the book is intended to be used by all health and mental health professionals, including social workers, psychologists, child care workers, physicians, physical and occupational therapists, and students who are interested in working collaboratively with their patients and clients.

Just a note of clarification: We use the terms *student* and *nurse* to pertain to both genders, male and female. Wherever possible, we have endeavoured to avoid using the feminine pronoun to refer to the nurse to acknowledge the increased number of males now entering this profession.

This book covers a wide range of topics on collaboration between the nurse and the person or family. Chapter 1 outlines what the collaborative partnership is and what distinguishes a collaborative approach from a traditional hierarchical approach. It also describes the historical and theoretical roots of collaboration and explains why collaboration is important today. In Chapter 2, the essential ingredients of a collaborative relationship are identified, including sharing of power, openness and respect, a nonjudgmental and accepting stance, the ability to tolerate ambiguity, and self-awareness and reflection. Chapter 3 describes the Spiralling Model of Collaborative Partnership, a four-phase process model that illustrates the establishment and progress of a collaborative relationship. Chapter 4 elaborates on the factors that shape the collaborative partnership, including nurse factors, person factors, relationship factors, and contextual or environmental factors. Chapter 5 highlights the specific strategies or behaviors that can be used by nurses in their practice to develop and maintain a collaborative partnership. Chapter 6 describes the key indicators that the nurse can look for in his or her own behaviour and the behaviour of the partner that indicate to what extent they are working together within this collaborative partnership framework. Finally, Chapters 7 and 8 consist of a series of questions posed to our panel of clinical nurse experts dealing with a range of issues and challenges related to the collaborative partnerships.

SUGGESTED READING

Gottlieb, L. N., & Ezer, H. (1997). *A Perspective on Health, Family, Learning, and Collaborative Nursing: A Collection of Writings on the McGill Model of Nursing*. Montreal: McGill University School of Nursing.

ACKNOWLEDGEMENTS

We wish to thank many people; without their encouragement and support this book would not have been written. First we wish to thank Dr. Susan French, director of McGill University School of Nursing, who suggested that a series of books on the various concepts of the McGill Model of Nursing be written. Dr. French is a person who not only comes up with ideas but also helps to make these ideas happen through her commitment of resources. These resources were made possible by the generosity of Richard and Satoko Ingram and the Newton Foundation. Richard and Satoko are committed to the development of excellence in nursing. They have been the prime movers in creating the impetus to help disseminate the ideas of the McGill nursing community to the larger nursing community.

We are indebted to Ann Millar, from Elsevier, who enthusiastically embraced this project and who has been our advocate, and to the anonymous reviewers for their excellent comments, which greatly improved the book. We are very grateful to Dawn du Quesnay, our developmental editor, for her perceptive comments and excellent suggestions throughout this process, and to Katherine Hinkebein, our project manager, who so skillfully shepherded us through the final stages. And special thanks go to Liz Radojkovic, with her keen eye for detail, who made important changes to the look of the book.

Thanks also go to Robin Canuel, Daniel Cassidy, and Raleen Murphy, who reviewed, retrieved, and organized the literature. Daniel Cassidy also transcribed the videotaped interviews with the nurse experts. Margie Gabriel coordinated the support staff. We also thank Marcia Beaulieu and Howard Richler, who clarified the terminology; and Daniel Heon, from the audiovisual department of the Montreal Children's Hospital, who videotaped the interviews.

REVIEWERS

Sandra Filice
Humber College
Toronto, Ontario

Anne Hofmeyer
University of Alberta
Edmonton, Alberta

Patricia Melanson
Dalhousie University
Halifax, Nova Scotia

Judith Shaw
St. Francis Xavier University
Antigonish, Nova Scotia

Jennifer Young
Red Deer College
Red Deer, Alberta

ABOUT THE AUTHORS

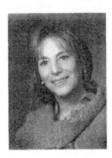

Laurie N. Gottlieb is a professor at the School of Nursing at McGill University and holds the Flora Madeline Shaw Chair of Nursing there. She is editor of the *CJNR (Canadian Journal of Nursing Research)*. She holds an M.Sc.(A) in nursing and a Ph.D. in developmental psychology. She participated in the original research on the McGill Model of Nursing and has researched, published, and extensively lectured on the model.

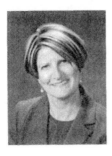

Nancy Feeley is an assistant professor at the McGill University School of Nursing and senior researcher at Sir Mortimer B. Davis Jewish General Hospital and project director at the Lady Davis Institute. Dr. Feeley holds an M.Sc.(A) and Ph.D. in nursing. She has research, nursing administration, and clinical experience with the McGill Model of Nursing. She teaches a graduate course on the use of the McGill Model of Nursing in practice.

Brief biographies follow of the nurses who made up our panel of expert clinicians. We thank them for sharing their knowledge and experience with us.

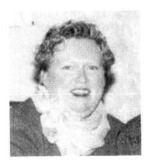

Jane Chambers-Evans, N. M.Sc.(A), M.Sc. (Bioethics), is a clinical nurse specialist in critical care and a clinical ethicist. She is also an assistant professor (part-time) at the McGill University School of Nursing and an affiliate to the Biomedical Ethics Unit, Faculty of Medicine, McGill University. Her clinical expertise is in the areas of family nursing, crisis intervention, grief counseling, and ethics. She works daily with patients, families, and a multidisciplinary team in the intensive care unit at the Montreal General Hospital site of the McGill University Health Centre. Her area of research is end-of-life decision making.

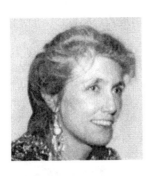

Joann Creager, N. M.Sc.(A), is a clinical nurse specialist in geriatrics and transition care at the Montreal General Hospital site of the McGill University Health Centre. Her clinical practice is with a geriatric clientele in both acute rehabilitation and long-term care settings, helping them and their families adjust effectively to functional and life changes. She also works with nursing staff on issues related to their practice and is particularly interested in end-of-life issues.

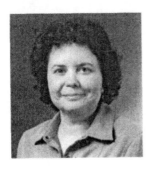

Cindy Dalton, N. M.Sc.(A), is a clinical nurse specialist in geriatrics at Sir Mortimer B. Davis Jewish General Hospital and a faculty lecturer (part-time) at the McGill University School of Nursing. She has also worked in neurology and in community health for many years. Her clinical interests include collaborative partnership and patients' readiness for change. As a faculty member, she developed and taught an undergraduate course on collaborative practice.

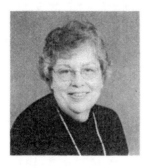

Margaret Eades, N. M.Sc.(A), is a clinical nurse specialist in oncology at the Montreal General Hospital site of the McGill University Health Centre and an assistant professor (part-time) at the McGill University School of Nursing. She works daily with patients and their families as they live the experience of cancer and is a teacher and mentor to staff nurses. Her area of research interest is the effect of activity on fatigue in cancer patients. She has been an active member of the Canadian Association of Nurses in Oncology for many years.

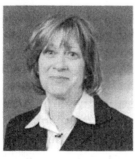

Lucia Fabijan, N. M.Sc.(A), is currently the nursing coordinator of Ambulatory Services, Neuroscience Mission, at McGill University Health Centre and is an assistant professor (part-time) at the McGill University School of Nursing. She teaches family assessment and intervention and is a clinical adviser for undergraduate and graduate students. She is a graduate of an accredited couple and family therapy training program and has a practice as a couple and family therapist. At the time of the interviews she was the Nursing Coordinator of External Services, Psychiatry, at the Sir Mortimer B. Davis Jewish General Hospital, where her responsibilities included leadership for advanced nursing practice in psychiatry, clinical practice with individuals with mental illnesses and their families, and teaching of psychosocial care, family nursing, and the therapeutic management of aggression.

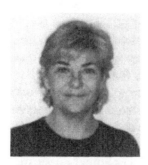

Catherine Pugnaire Gros, N. M.Sc.(A), is a faculty lecturer at the McGill University School of Nursing, where she has taught graduate and undergraduate students since 1985. She is also a clinical nurse specialist in mental health at the Douglas Hospital. The focus of her work as an educator, clinician, and researcher has been on the development and clinical application of collaborative, family-centred practice.

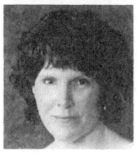

Heather D. Hart, B.Ed., B.Sc.N., M.Sc.(A), is a staff nurse working in palliative care (adult patient population) within the McGill University Health Centre. She has served as a clinical teacher for nursing students both in palliative care and geriatric settings, and she lectures at the McGill University School of Nursing.

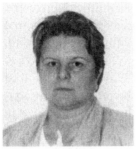

Irène Leboeuf, M.Sc.N., is currently a clinical nurse specialist in pediatric hemato-oncology at Ste. Justine Hospital. At the time of the interviews she was working in adult neuro-oncology as a clinical nurse specialist at the Montreal Neurological Hospital of the McGill University Health Centre. Her clinical interests are oncology, support groups for patients with brain tumours and their families, and family systems nursing.

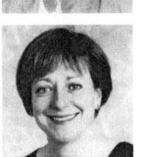

Diane Lowden, N. M.Sc.(A), is a multiple sclerosis certified nurse and a clinical nurse specialist in the Multiple Sclerosis Program at the Montreal Neurological Hospital of the McGill University Health Centre. She is also an assistant professor (part-time) at the McGill University School of Nursing. As an advanced practice nurse, she works with individuals and families around issues related to coping with multiple sclerosis (MS). Ms. Lowden is a member of the Canadian MS Nurses Network and the International Organization of Multiple Sclerosis Nurses. She collaborates regularly with these groups on initiatives around clinical care, education, and research, and she lectures nationally and internationally to professional groups on the care of individuals with MS and their families.

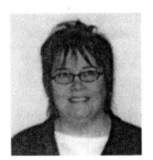

Deborah Radford-Moudarres, B.Sc.N., M.Sc.(A), is currently employed by Chenango County–Harry Stack Sullivan Mental Health Services in New York State as a psychiatric nurse practitioner intern. She also cofacilitates an anxiety management group. She is currently enrolled in a program for post–master's certification as a psychiatric/mental health nurse practitioner at the University of New York, Stony Brook. At the time of the interviews she worked at the Sir Mortimer B. Davis Jewish General Hospital as a clinical nurse specialist in outpatient psychiatry.

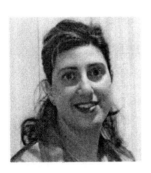

Rosalia (Lia) Sanzone, B.Sc.N., M.Sc.(A), is acting coordinator of the Maternal-Child-Family Program at CLSC Métro. She has worked since 1990 at CLSC Métro, which has a multicultural population, with families in school health and perinatality. She has also been a course lecturer at the McGill University School of Nursing since 2001.

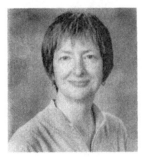

Gillian Taylor, N. M.Sc.(A), is a clinical nurse specialist (CNS) in ambulatory services at the Montreal Children's Hospital of the McGill University Health Centre, working in rheumatology, and is a faculty lecturer (part-time) at the McGill University School of Nursing. In her role as a CNS, she provides care, education, and support to families of children with chronic rheumatic conditions, and she liaises with community health services and schools. She is involved at the provincial and national levels in the promotion of the needs of young people with juvenile arthritis within the networks of organizations working to raise awareness and research funds for arthritis.

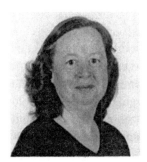

Jackie Townshend, N. M.Sc.(A), at the time of the interviews was nurse-coordinator for the Cystic Fibrosis Clinic of the Montreal Children's Hospital at the McGill University Health Centre. In this role, she nursed children from birth to 18 years of age and families living with the challenges of a hereditary, life-limiting, chronic illness and acted as the coordinator of the multidisciplinary team. She is currently enjoying the quiet life in Nova Scotia and works as a volunteer at a home for the elderly.

CONTENTS

PART II: ASK THE EXPERTS

The

COLLABORATIVE PARTNERSHIP APPROACH TO CARE

A Delicate Balance

Part

I

THE COLLABORATIVE PARTNERSHIP

Chapter 1

FOUNDATIONS OF COLLABORATIVE PARTNERSHIP

Collaboration means seeing what the client and their family members have as goals for their health, and working with them, enlisting their help, providing my expertise, and finding a way that we can work together to get to achieve those goals.

—Nurse Joann Creager

After reading this chapter you should be able to:
- Describe two basic forms of the nurse-person relationship and the features of each
- Define a collaborative partnership
- State the 10 principles of collaborative partnership
- Identify and describe the six forces that have influenced the need for nurses to adopt a collaborative partnership approach
- Describe the evidence that a collaborative partnership approach is effective

The term *collaboration* has worked its way into our everyday lexicon in the health care arena. It is a term that typically conjures up images of something progressive, something positive. It is a term that has been extended to describe the nature of the relationship between the health professional and the person. *Partnership* is another familiar term that is often used interchangeably with *collaboration*. In this book we have combined these two words. We use *collaboration* as the adjective to describe the desired nature of the nurse-person partnership, hence the term *collaborative partnership*.

This book is about the collaborative partnership between the nurse and the person. The ideas, principles, and guidelines presented here can apply to any health care provider and person relationship, but we focus on the nurse-person relationship because nurses have been particularly sensitive to this relationship.

In fact, the nurse-person relationship is considered central to nursing practice, and it is through this relationship that nursing is experienced and expressed.

We have chosen to use the word *person* rather than *patient* or *client* because the word *patient* usually refers to the role a person assumes in hospital or when sick, and the word *client* is a term that has been adopted by nurses working with "healthy" individuals in the community. When we use the word *person* we are in fact referring to the other partner in the collaborative partnership; this partner could be an individual, a family, a community, or any other aggregate group or population with whom the nurse is involved. The word *person* is encompassing, neutral, not tied to place or role, and carries fewer negative connotations than the alternatives.

Pioneering nursing scholars such as Peplau (1952) and Orlando (1961) understood that the nature of the nurse-person relationship was at the heart of helping people become healthier and deal with and manage life events, illness, trauma, injuries, and death. Even nursing interventions that are primarily technical in nature are viewed as an interpersonal event involving the nurse and the person. It is this legacy that has made the nurse-person relationship the central feature of nursing. There are different ways of conceptualizing or viewing the nurse-person relationship, and each gives rise to a different approach to nursing. The two basic forms of the nurse-person relationship are the *traditional hierarchical* and the *collaborative partnership*.

TRADITIONAL HIERARCHICAL RELATIONSHIPS VS. COLLABORATIVE PARTNERSHIPS

The **traditional hierarchical relationship** has been the dominant form within nursing as well as within most of the helping professions. The traditional hierarchical approach has also been referred to as the *authoritative, paternalistic approach,* the *unilateral relationship,* and the *professional model of practice.* The traditional hierarchical relationship has emerged from an illness-treatment legacy in which the health professional assumed the role of the expert who had the knowledge and power to treat and cure disease. This form of the nurse-person relationship is rooted in an ethos of caring based on a paternalistic system of values. This system of values shares many of the same characteristics as the parent-child relationship in which the parent is the health care professional and the child is the person. In a paternalistic system of values, one partner in the relationship (the professional or the "parent") is considered to possess the knowledge and expertise and thus "knows best." The professional assumes the authority and power to make decisions and assumes responsibility for the person's health. The role of the person, in exchange for being taken care of, is to comply with the professional's plan.

An alternative form of the professional-person relationship is the collaborative partnership that has emerged from the health promotion movement. Other approaches that have similar features include *reciprocal relationships, self-determination relationships, participatory practices,* and *mutual relationships.*

Collaborative partnership is rooted in an ethos of caring based on an egalitarian system of values. This system shares many of the same characteristics as an adult-adult relationship in which each partner has comparable status and power (Lowenberg, 1989; McQueen, 2000). In an egalitarian system of values, the professional's role is to help the other person in the relationship grow and develop (Mayeroff, 1972) and to support the person's efforts to make decisions and assume responsibility for his own health. Both partners in the relationship are considered to have knowledge and expertise, albeit of a different type. The partners exhibit mutual respect for one another, and the relationship is mutually beneficial to both parties because both grow and develop through their involvement in this relationship (Halstead, Wagner, Margo, & Ferkol, 2002).

The traditional hierarchical and the collaborative partnership forms of the nurse-person relationship differ in a number of ways: their underlying assumptions, the focus of care, the role of the nurse, the role of the person, the nature of the relationship, how goals are determined, the nature of evaluation, and the expected outcomes. Table 1-1 summarizes how the features of each of these compare to one another.

The key feature of the traditional hierarchical relationship is that the professionals view themselves as experts who have the knowledge to determine what is best for the "uninformed" person. This knowledge provides the professionals with the power base for setting goals, making decisions, and finding solutions to problems. In contrast, the collaborative partnership relationship is predicated on the professionals viewing themselves as possessing expert knowledge while at the same time recognizing that the person has unique knowledge that is critical to the decision-making and planning process of care.

The other key feature that distinguishes between these two forms of the nurse-person relationship is how decisions are made. In the traditional hierarchical relationship, decisions are made primarily by the professional, whereas in the collaborative partnership relationship, the decisions and evaluations are the joint responsibility of both partners. This requires each partner (i.e., both the nurse and the person) to consider the other partner's perceptions, needs, and goals in order to achieve a delicate balance. Finally, in the collaborative partnership, both the professional and the person learn, gain, and grow from the relationship.

THE PHILOSOPHICAL STANCE UNDERLYING THE COLLABORATIVE PARTNERSHIP

When nurses adopt a collaborative partnership approach to care, they are subscribing to a certain set of beliefs, values, and attitudes about people, nursing, and the nurse-person relationship. Some refer to this set of beliefs, values, and attitudes as a philosophical stance. A **philosophical stance** suggests *how* the nurse should interact and work with people and is reflected in every

TABLE 1-1	Traditional Hierarchical vs. Collaborative Partnership Forms of the Nurse-Person Relationship	
Comparison Criteria	**Traditional Hierarchical (Paternalism)**	**Collaborative Partnership**
Assumptions	The person needs to be taken care of by the professional. The person is passive and not responsible for his care. The person lacks knowledge or the capabilities to understand and manage his illness or problems. The professional possesses the knowledge and capabilities to manage illness and problems. The professional has the control and responsibility.	The person is active and shares responsibility for his care. The person has knowledge and capabilities that he can use to understand and manage his illness or problems or work toward his goals in ways that are meaningful to him.
Focus	The person's illness, symptoms, or problems.	The person's ability to be well, experience a high quality of life, and live in a meaningful way.
Role of nurse	The expert who holds the knowledge and, thus, solves problems and makes decisions.	A facilitator who encourages people to share their perceptions and expertise, to participate in joint decision making, and to develop the person's autonomy (i.e., ability to be self-directed) and self-efficacy. Helps people more fully use their strengths and resources. Has knowledge of their illnesses and themselves.
Role of person	A passive recipient of professional's expertise.	An active partner who plays an important role in setting goals and finding solutions that best fit the person.
Nature of relationship	Is characterized by the professional in the dominant role and the person in the subordinate role. There is a differential of power, and the relationship is asymmetrical.	Is reciprocal and mutual; each partner gives and receives and, thus, the relationship is more symmetrical or balanced. Involves the continual negotiation of goals, roles, and responsibilities. Both partners give up some autonomy as they value and trust the other's expertise. Both partners gain and grow.
Goal setting	Professional determines the goals, typically based on the problem only.	Goals are jointly determined.

(Continued)

TABLE 1-1 Traditional Hierarchical vs. Collaborative Partnership Forms of the Nurse-Person Relationship		
Comparison Criteria	**Traditional Hierarchical (Paternalism)**	**Collaborative Partnership**
Evaluation	Professional assesses progress in achieving her goals for the person.	The partners share in joint assessment of progress in achieving mutually determined goals.
Expected outcome	The problem is solved or the person is considered noncompliant, thereby possibly being blamed for an unsuccessful outcome.	The problem may or may not be solved but the person's capabilities to manage current or future problems are enhanced. Joint responsibility is accepted for the outcomes.

Based on a synthesis of the ideas of Allen, 1977; Courtney, Ballard, Fauver, Gariota, & Holland, 1996; Gottlieb, 1997; Gottlieb & Rowat, 1997; Hall & Allan, 1994; Kasch, 1986; and Pratto & Walker, 2001.

interaction and in every encounter. The nurse's beliefs, values, and attitudes that underlie the collaborative partnership relate to how power is shared between the nurse and the person, how decisions are made, how care is planned, each person's respective roles, and how each partner relates to the other.

At the beginning of this book, in the section Our Panel of Experts, we introduced a number of expert nurse clinicians who shared their experiences with us. From time to time, we will relate their experiences to illustrate the application of the theory in this text. When asked for her views on collaboration, for example, Nurse Gillian Taylor, who works with children who have arthritis and their families, explained, *"To me collaboration is a stance that I take—a place that I put myself in—which says 'I don't know what's best. I have a lot of knowledge, and I have biases, and I have goals, and I have hopes for persons and families.' But my collaborative stance says, 'I don't know where I'm going to go.' It doesn't take away from the fact that I'm active and I have lots to bring to the relationship and the work that gets done, but it's a stance that says, 'I don't know how this will come together.' It also means that as a nurse I will pay a lot of attention to the relationship with the family and person or client. Where they're going to go . . . or how they should be, or what they should do, that is also important. A collaborative approach says, 'I will pay attention to the relationship with these people.'"*

THE COLLABORATIVE PARTNERSHIP: A DEFINITION

In the literature, the terms *partnership* and *collaboration* are often used interchangeably. In a concept analysis of the nurse-person partnership, Gallant, Beaulieu, and Carnevale (2002) reviewed more than 100 articles from the nursing, medicine, social sciences, and psychology literature. They defined partnership as "an interpersonal relationship between two or more people who work together toward a mutually defined purpose" (p. 151). McQueen (2000) synthesized the nursing literature on the meaning of partnership and defined nursing partnerships as "an association between nurse and patient where each one is a respected, autonomous individual with something to contribute to a joint venture, and in which both work towards an agreed goal" (p. 726).

We define **collaborative partnership** as the pursuit of person-centred goals through a dynamic process that requires the active participation and agreement of all partners. The relationship is one of partnership and the way of working together is collaborative, hence the term *collaborative partnership*. The features of a collaborative partnership are as follows:

- Power sharing and sharing of expertise
- Pursuit of mutually agreed-on, person-centred goals
- Creation of a dynamic process that requires the active participation and agreement of all partners in the relationship

We now examine each of these three features in greater detail.

Power Sharing in the Collaborative Partnership

Power sharing is the hallmark of collaborative partnership. In a collaborative partnership relationship, the agenda and goals of both the person and the nurse are given hearing and importance (Kasch, 1986). All participants bring something (i.e., knowledge, experience, expertise) to the relationship. The nurse recognizes and values the abilities, knowledge, skills, and experience of the other person. It is this recognition by the nurse of the person's expertise that serves as the leverage for the person's power. Kasch noted that a collaborative nurse-person relationship may require that the person take on new roles to engage in decision making and problem solving with the nurse to determine goals and weigh alternative courses of action.

Nurse Lucia Fabijan who works with people who are mentally ill stated that *"collaboration means understanding who the person is and what he wishes to discuss and share and what he would like to change or accomplish in his own life. The agenda for work derives from the person in front of you. The agenda for work is not nurse driven."*

Nurse Jane Chambers-Evans, who works in an intensive care unit, elaborated on the idea that the collaborative partnership is a partnership of two actively involved parties: *"To me you can't collaborate if there aren't partners—that is, if only one of you is doing the work and the other's only contribution is to try and keep you away. I don't see that as collaboration. I don't see it as collaboration until there's been some kind of engagement."*

The Focus on Mutually Agreed-On, Person-Centred Goals

Generally collaboration is thought of as two or more people working together in pursuit of a common goal (DeChillo, Koren, & Schultze, 1994; Kim, 1983; Williamson, 1981). The Comox Valley Nursing Centre (Clarke & Mass, 1998) developed this definition of collaboration for nursing practice: "Collaboration is a joint communicating and decision-making process with the expressed goal of satisfying the client's wellness and illness needs while respecting the unique qualities and abilities of the client and the nurse" (p. 18). Our definition of collaborative partnership includes this notion of the nurse and person working toward goals that are mutually determined.

Nurse Joann Creager who works with elderly patients in hospital explained: *"Collaboration, to me, means that I am trying to see what the client and their family members have as goals for their health. I'm working with them, enlisting their help, providing my expertise, and finding a way that we can work together to achieve those goals. And in some cases I may have goals in mind that they may not have thought of, so I might share those goals with them to see if they're appropriate goals to work on."*

Collaboration as a Dynamic Process

We view the collaborative partnership as a process that takes place between the nurse and person. It is similar to the phases of the nursing process or the problem-solving process. The process is dynamic inasmuch as it requires the active participation and agreement of all partners. It has different phases and different subprocesses including exchanging information, establishing trust, negotiating, and prioritizing goals. The phases of the collaborative partnership are elaborated in Chapter 3.

COOPERATION AND PATIENT PARTICIPATION: RELATED CONCEPTS

Cooperation is just a first step toward the more complex process of collaborative partnership. **Cooperation** is defined as "planning and working together in a helpful way" (Baggs & Schmitt, 1988). A person can be unassertive, passive, and yet cooperative. Cooperation should not be confused with collaboration. Cooperation is a prerequisite for a collaborative partnership; that is to say collaboration requires some measure of cooperation. However, it also involves assertiveness and active involvement. Not all acts of cooperation are acts of collaboration, but all acts of collaboration require cooperation.

Participation means that the person gets involved at some level or is allowed to be involved in the decision-making process or the delivery of a service (Brearley, 1990). Person participation or involvement can be viewed on a continuum that progresses from the passive person and the active health professional through the more active person and less active professional to the stage where the level of activity approaches equality and, finally, to a stage where the person is active and the health professional is inactive. The optimum balance between person and professional activity depends on the type of health problem, the person's preference and potential for participation, and the situational context (Brearley, 1990).

An alternative way of thinking about person participation is in terms of different ways persons participate in their care. Klein (as cited in Biley, 1992) has described five distinct categories of participation:

1. *Information:* For some, participation means that the professional gives the person information and the person's role is to receive it.
2. *Consultation:* For others, the term participation refers to the professional consulting the person and then perhaps using the information gained to plan the person's care.
3. *Negotiation:* In this case, there is greater participation between the professional and the person and negotiations take place between the two.
4. *Participation:* Both the professional and the person share in the decision making.
5. *Veto participation:* The person has the power or the right to veto any care decisions.

We consider negotiation, participation, and veto participation (where either partner has veto power) to be the classes of participation that best fit our view of collaborative partnership. Thus, what person participation has in common with collaborative partnership is that the person is central to the decision-making process and is an active, involved participant.

PRINCIPLES OF THE COLLABORATIVE PARTNERSHIP

We have identified 10 major principles that underlie the collaborative partnership:

1. Both person and nurse want to and agree to enter into a collaborative relationship.
2. The collaborative partnership can assume many forms depending on the person's preferences, abilities, and circumstances.
3. The nurse continuously assesses the conditions that influence collaboration and adjusts the form that the collaborative partnership takes to best fit the person's needs and abilities and the situation.
4. The collaborative partnership is purposeful and goal directed.

5. To achieve mutually agreed-on goals, both the nurse and the person need to have as thorough an understanding of the situation as is possible at that point in time. This involves sharing with one another the other's unique perspective.
6. In a collaborative partnership, the person is the essential and primary source of information.
7. Both person and nurse contribute resources that are used collaboratively.
8. Collaboration, in some situations, involves sharing a very different perspective with a person, challenging his view, or inviting him to see something different.
9. The collaborative partnership may change within an encounter and across encounters as the situation changes or as the person's needs or abilities evolve.
10. A collaborative partnership approach requires a varied repertoire of communication and interpersonal skills.

WHY COLLABORATIVE PARTNERSHIP IS IMPORTANT TODAY: THE SIX FORCES

During the past few decades there has been a growing awareness that a collaborative approach to care is both desirable and necessary (Coulter, 1999; Patterson, 1995). Changes in society and health care services have prompted this reexamination of the traditional hierarchical professional-person relationship and the need for an alternative approach to care.

In this section, we describe six forces that have contributed to the support for a collaborative partnership approach within the health care systems of many countries such as Australia, Canada, the United Kingdom, and the United States to name just a few. These six forces are as follows:

1. Consumerism and patient rights
2. Primary health care and health promotion
3. Accessibility of health information
4. Changes in thinking about nursing and ethical care
5. Shift from hospital-based to home-based care
6. Current knowledge about how people change

Force 1: Consumerism and Patient Rights

The idea that health care professionals should view persons as partners came to the forefront during the late 1960s and early 1970s with the growth of the consumer movement. Consumers began to question how they were being treated in both service and professional industries, and this questioning extended to the health care system and people's rights as patients (Biley, 1992; Cahill, 1998; Kirk & Glendinning, 1998; McQueen, 2000; Sullivan, 1998). Concomitant with the public wanting to assume greater responsibility and power in determining its care (Lowenberg, 1989), the public began to evaluate its role and the role of its health providers. As people became more knowledgeable and confident in their own abilities to make decisions, they began to question the paternalistic "I-know-best" attitude that predominated the behaviour of health care professionals.

The need for a collaborative approach to care has taken on greater relevancy in recent years as a result of health care fiscal constraints and changes in the way health care is delivered (Cahill, 1998). During the 1980s and 1990s, the spiraling costs of health care services prompted health care administrators and policy makers to find solutions to contain health care costs. This has led to increased tension between health care consumers and those who manage and determine the nature of health care services, whether governments, as in the case of Canada, or other organizations, such as health maintenance organizations in the United States. This tension has led to a return to more person-centred care as well as a desire to educate consumers about the costs of health care and help them learn how to be more judicious and knowledgeable users of these services (Sullivan, 1998). It is believed that health care can be provided more efficiently and effectively if people participate in the decision-making and implementation of their own health care (Hollman & Lorig, 2000).

Force 2: Primary Health Care and Health Promotion Principles

Increasing evidence that early childhood experiences and lifestyle choices are major determinants of long-term morbidity and mortality has led to the need to consider allocating more resources to health promotion and illness prevention. The desire to shift our health care system's focus from illness to health has resulted in accelerated acceptance and growth in primary health care and health promotion movements in recent years. One of the five key principles of primary health care outlined by the World Health Organization (WHO) was client participation in care (cited in MacIntosh & McCormack, 2001). WHO has also defined health promotion as "the process of enabling people to increase control over and improve their health" (cited in Strickland & Strickland, 1996, p. 22). A key underlying premise of primary health care is collaboration between professionals and people (Stewart, 1990). Canadian nurses Young and Hayes (2002) have described a transformative approach to health promotion in nursing that is based on a collaborative process in which health professionals work with individuals, families, communities, and populations to take action to improve health. It has been argued that the best way to involve people in their own care is for the professional to develop a collaborative partnership with the people for whom they care (Strickland & Strickland, 1996). It is believed that when people collaborate in their own health care it is more likely that their care will be customized to meet their needs (MacIntosh & McCormack, 2001). It is also more likely that they will feel more satisfied with their care because they have a greater sense of control over their health. Finally, they are more likely to follow the treatment plan because they participated in its development (Roberts & Krouse, 1988).

Force 3: Access to Health Information

The growth of telecommunications has altered the way in which people relate to health care providers. Health information is more readily available via the Internet, television, and radio, and this availability has been influential in promoting people's desire and ability to participate in their care. In fact, the Information Superhighway has changed the fundamental way people are relating to and interacting with health care providers (Loiselle & Dubois, 2003). We have a well-informed public that expects a greater say in its own care. In the past, knowledge was the sole purview of the health care professional. Today people have better education and access to information they want. They now need health professionals who can help them sort, decipher, locate, and interpret the information relevant to them.

Force 4: Current Thinking about Nursing and Ethical Nursing Care

Involving people in their care is now a widely accepted principle underlying contemporary nursing practice. Thus, another force that has given rise to collaborative approaches to nursing care is the current philosophy of nursing that has moved toward patient-centred care and patient participation in care (Cahill, 1998). Primary nursing (i.e., when one nurse assumes responsibility for the patient's care) as a method of organizing nursing care has also prompted a shift from the nurse as a distant professional to that of the individual responsible for the patient's individualized, holistic care (Kirk & Glendinning, 1998; McQueen, 2000). Thus, changes within the discipline of nursing itself have been important in giving rise to nurses' adoption of collaborative approaches to care.

Professional associations have codes of ethical conduct to guide professionals' practice and behaviour. These codes of ethics reflect the profession's underlying beliefs and values about people, the profession, and the relationship between the two. For example, the Canadian Nurses Association (1997) has identified eight key values that are central to nursing practice. Two central values are choice/autonomy and dignity/respect, and these values call for nurses to use a collaborative approach in caring for persons and families.

- *Choice/autonomy:* Nurses should respect and promote the autonomy of people. Thus, nurses seek to involve people in health planning and health decision making. Nurses should provide the support that people require to act on their own behalf to meet their health care needs. Nurses should also be sensitive to their position of relative power in the relationship and purposefully promote their partner's self-determination. Nurses should seek to involve all people, even those of diminished competence, in decision making to the extent to which they are capable.
- *Dignity/respect:* Nurses should recognize and respect the inherent worth of each person. Nurses should be sensitive to people's individual needs, values, and choices; this sensitivity reflects their respect for the person. Nurses should respect people by trying to understand and support people's desired quality of life and wishes.

Force 5: The Shift from Hospital to Home-Based Care

With the shift from hospital to ambulatory care, the increasing prevalence of chronic conditions, the aging population, and the need to control health care costs, care of the person has for the most part shifted to the family as caregivers (Cahill, 1996, 1998; Hollman & Lorig, 2000; Kirk, 2001). Therefore, for people to be able to effectively manage their own care or that of their family members, they need to be knowledgeable about the condition and treatment and must play a central role in devising the plan of care; otherwise, the plan is doomed. This has required a reconceptualization of the health care professional-family relationship. A collaborative partnership better prepares the person and family to these responsibilities better than a traditional hierarchical relationship would.

Force 6: Knowledge of How People Change

Most health and illness situations require that people change their behaviours or lifestyles. People have knowledge that is important to decision making concerning their care. Some people who live with a chronic condition have greater knowledge about their condition and more expertise in managing it than do many professionals. People also possess important information about themselves and their own personal preferences that is critical to planning their care. People need to be involved in the process of altering their behaviour if they are going to make long-lasting behavioural changes.

We know that effective behavioural change requires that people play the primary role in determining the need for change and designing a plan for change (Westberg & Jason, 1996). People are more likely to work toward goals that they set for themselves rather than those set by someone else (Carey, 1989). They are also more likely to be accountable for decisions that they make than those made by others. Thus, professionals can be most helpful in helping people change their behaviour when they facilitate and encourage the person's process of change and act as a coach or consultant rather than the expert who tells them what to do and how to do it.

Box 1-1 summarizes the six forces behind the collaborative partnership.

Box 1-1	The Six Forces Behind the Collaborative Partnership

- Consumerism and patient rights
- Primary health care and health promotion
- Accessibility of health information
- Changes in thinking about nursing and ethical care
- Shift from hospital-based to home-based care
- Current knowledge about how people change

IS A COLLABORATIVE APPROACH EFFECTIVE?

Evidence-based nursing involves considering multiple sources of evidence from research, clinical expertise, and patient preferences into decisions about the health care of individual persons (MulHall, 1998). Our nursing decisions should be based on sound evidence and the best available evidence that we have to practice as well as we can (Estabrooks, 1998). Nursing practice is derived from many different ways of knowing. Nurses draw on ethical knowledge, personal knowledge, empirical knowledge, and aesthetical knowledge (Carper, 1978; James & Lorentzon, 2004). These different ways of knowing require different forms of evidence on which to base best practice decisions. These forms range from the randomized control trial to qualitative studies, descriptive studies, case studies, and autobiographical accounts (Smith, 2004).

What evidence do we have that a collaborative partnership approach to practice is effective? Effectiveness can be assessed in a number of ways. We need to consider, for example, whether people are more satisfied with the care they receive when their relationship with professionals is collaborative than when it is not. Do people describe their health as "better" if they are working collaboratively with professionals? Do people feel more in control of their health care when they work collaboratively with professionals? Do people want to participate in a collaborative partnership with professionals? What do people who have experienced a collaborative partnership say about this approach? What do professionals say about this approach? Is it useful and in what ways?

Several studies have examined these very questions. Note that many of these studies have examined other professionals' adoption of a collaborative approach to care, not that of nurses. Roberts and Krouse (1989) conducted an experimental study to assess the effectiveness of a collaborative approach to nursing practice based on their model of an actively negotiated process of nurse-person decision making. They used simulated nurse-person encounters rather than actual encounters, and nursing students role-played the roles of person and nurse. Participants who experienced an actively negotiated process of decision making with the "nurse" about their treatment reported feeling more in control than participants who experienced a partial negotiation or nonnegotiation approach concerning their treatment.

A meta-analysis of 41 studies of physician-person relationships found that when physicians engaged in partnership building with their patients by eliciting their input and when assuming a less controlling or dominant role, patients were more satisfied with their care (Hall, Roter, & Katz, 1988). Similarly, in a study of ambulatory psychiatric patients (Eisenthal & Lazare, 1976), when psychiatrists, psychologists, and social workers used a "customer" approach (i.e., akin to collaborative partnership approach), patients reported being more satisfied with their care, felt better, and were more likely to feel that their care was what they hoped for.

People who work collaboratively with health professionals experience better health and well-being. Greenfield and colleagues (1988) conducted an interesting series of studies to determine if they could increase patient participation in their care. While ambulatory patients with diabetes were waiting to see their physicians, they were taught how to ask questions and how to negotiate care decisions with the physicians. The researchers found that patients who applied the skills and were actively involved in decision making with their physicians subsequently had better blood sugar control, reported higher quality of life, knew more about diabetes, and were more satisfied with their care. When the same study was repeated with patients suffering from ulcers, similar results were obtained (Greenfield, Kaplan, & Ware, 1985). They also found that not every patient was able to take the ideas that they were given during the brief teaching session and become involved in their care. However, people who participated the most in decision making had the best blood sugar control. This suggests that if patients living with diabetes are more passive in their care, their passivity might jeopardize their ability to control their disease, thereby putting them at greater risk for complications of diabetes. The Greenfield studies teach us two important lessons. First, people who are partners in their care with professionals may be better able to manage their care and, thus, may experience better health outcomes. Second, people can be taught to become partners in their own care.

Not only do adults benefit from this approach but children also benefit either directly or indirectly when their parents work collaboratively with a nurse. In a randomized controlled trial of a yearlong nursing intervention based on the McGill Model of Nursing in which a collaborative partnership was the form of the nurse-person relationship, children living with chronic conditions who received the intervention experienced better psychosocial adjustment compared to children who received routine care (Pless et al., 1994).

DO PEOPLE WANT TO PARTICIPATE IN A COLLABORATIVE PARTNERSHIP WITH PROFESSIONALS?

Those who subscribe to a collaborative partnership approach to care make the assumption that people want to work collaboratively with professionals. A number of studies have questioned the validity of this assumption and cite evidence from studies to conclude that many people prefer professionals telling them what to do rather than having a say in the decision-making process. Note that many of these studies were done in the 1980s when health care professionals' behaviour and people's expectations about their role in their care may have been quite different from today.

The first study is by Strull and colleagues (1984) who asked ambulatory persons with high blood pressure who should make decisions about medication to treat their condition. Forty-seven percent of respondents thought that the physician should make the decision, 31% thought the professional should make the decision but take into consideration the person's opinion, 19% thought both should share equally in the decision, 2% thought the person should decide while considering the professional's opinion, and 1% thought that the person alone should decide. Although these results have been used as evidence that people do not want to collaborate with health professionals, these results could also indicate that, although many people with high blood pressure may not want to decide what medication they should be prescribed, this does not preclude their wanting to be involved in other decisions about their medications. For example, the person who decides that his physician should make the decision about which medication to be prescribed may want, on the other hand, to have a say in when the medication should be taken. Another possibility is that, as Brearley (1990) suggests, when persons are asked whether they want to participate they respond in the negative because they have never experienced this type of relationship. People tend to "prefer" that which is familiar and known.

Another study that is often cited to support the argument for a traditional hierarchical approach to care rather than a collaborative approach is the study by

Waterworth and Luker (1990). Twelve hospitalized patients were asked how they were involved in decisions about their nursing care, and most indicated that they were not interested in participating in decisions. Rather, they just wanted to "stay out of trouble" by behaving in ways the nurses expected them to behave, so they followed the routine and "toed the line." The findings of this study do not really answer the question of whether people *want* to be partners in their care. However, the findings do suggest that the nursing or organizational culture of a unit might play a large role in affecting whether or not people are treated as partners in their own care (Trnobranski, 1994). A more recent study of hospitalized Finnish patients found that whereas 35% of patients agreed that nursing staff should make decisions about treatment, 65% disagreed (Suhonen, Valimaki, & Katajisto, 2000). We need to remember that people may have varying levels of desire and ability to participate as partners in their own care (Allen, 2000).

Many factors affect to what extent people want to be involved in making decisions about their care, such as how they are feeling, what knowledge is required to make the decision, and whether they feel comfortable assuming responsibility for the decision. In Chapter 4 of this book, we present a framework that identifies the various people, nurse, and environment factors that might influence the collaborative partnership. A case in point is the study by Biley (1992), which showed that many factors influenced surgical patients' participation in decisions about their care while in hospital. Patients perceived that their participation varied according to their physical condition. When patients were acutely ill, they were willing to let nurses make decisions regarding their care. However, as patients began to recover, their desire for involvement in decision making increased. Patients also perceived that the information needed to make a decision affected their desire to be involved in decision making. When they did not have information, patients felt that the nurse should make the decisions. This occurred most frequently with regard to medical or technical decisions, such as when to do dressing changes. In other situations, such as performing activities of daily living, patients felt that they had sufficient information and wanted to have their say. The question "Do people want to collaborate?" is really too simplistic. The question that needs to be asked is "How do people want to collaborate, around what issues, in what situations and settings, and at what point in time?"

According to the people interviewed by Thorne and Robinson (1988), people prefer to delegate some care decisions to professionals. This is consistent with the observation that although people may say they want to decide on their treatment, when faced with cancer they will frequently ask the physician to make the decisions about treatment (Brink, 1992). In a similar vein, Thompson and colleagues (1993) studied patients' desires to be involved in decisions about their medical treatment. They found that patients expressed a desire to be involved in decisions that did not require medical expertise, but were less likely to want to be involved in decisions that required medical knowledge. Some elderly hospitalized patients who believed that they should not play an active role in making decisions about their care cited the following reasons: The health care professionals "were the experts," they "knew best," and "it's naturally better to take their advice" (Roberts, 2002, p. 86). This suggests that the nature of the decision and the knowledge required to make that decision may be key to whether people want to make decisions about their care.

It would appear that what is critical in a collaborative approach to care is that the person has a say in who is the best person(s) to make a decision in any given situation. For example, in a collaborative approach, the professional and the person may together decide that the professional is the best person to make a decision about a treatment option, whereas they may decide that the person is best suited to decide on lifestyle options. When people have been asked by the professional to make a decision and then ask the professional to make that decision for them, they have in essence made the decision. Moreover, this process is quite different from never being asked to decide (Brink, 1992). A study by De Ridder and colleagues (1997) suggests that many persons want to act as responsible decision makers concerning their health care if health care professionals create an environment in which persons are given guidance in determining their alternatives.

Kirschbaum and Knafl (1996) studied 52 families who had a child with a chronic or critical condition and found three patterns of how families wanted to be involved in the decision-making process involving their child's care. The first pattern was called "Dependent." Parents in this group preferred to play a more passive role in their child's care and put their trust in health care providers to make decisions for them. The second pattern was called "Independent Decision Making." These parents viewed themselves as competent decision makers and the professional as a consultant whose advice they could either accept or reject. They valued professional input as potentially useful, but also trusted their own abilities. They expected professionals to be respectful of their decisions and their ability to make decisions. The third pattern was called "Collaborative Decision Makers." This group of parents had developed expertise in making decisions about their child's care. They described their relationship with the professional as being based on mutual respect. They valued the professional's input yet also knew the importance of their own perspective. They worked collaboratively with professionals to negotiate how best to incorporate the professional's input. They used the word *we* to describe how decisions were made together with professionals.

In fact, when people want to collaborate but are not given the opportunity to share in decision making with health professionals, they experience feelings of frustration and anger and their relationship with the professional can be seriously undermined. Families with a chronically ill child and families with an adult member with cancer participated in a study that examined the relationships families had with health care professionals (Robinson & Thorne, 1984). When families first became involved with professionals, they expected to share in decision making about care. However, when professionals withheld information, did not value the family's perspective, and expected the family to passively comply with their plan for the family, then families experienced feelings of anger and frustration and the family's relationship with the professional deteriorated. Patterson (2001) also found that Canadian adults living with diabetes wanted to work with professionals as partners in their care, but noted that professionals discounted the adults' experiential knowledge and did not provide them with the information that they needed to make decisions about their care. In a similar vein, two studies from the United Kingdom found that family members reported wanting to be involved in the care of their sick family member in hospital, but found it difficult to do so because health professionals would not enter into negotiations over how they could (Allen, 2000; Kirk, 2001).

Overall the results of these studies suggest that while not everyone wants to collaborate in decision making around their own care at all times, many people do. Variations are certain to exist among people. There is a continuum of collaboration and every person has a level of operating at which he is most comfortable. Moreover, within each person, the level of collaboration may vary depending on the situation, the circumstance, and the time. In some situations, people may want to maintain full control over decision making and in other situations they may want to share decision making with the professional, and in yet others they may want to relinquish control to the professional. We fully agree with Dennis's (1990) conclusion that "it would seem important for nurses to support persons who want to be included in decision making, yet relieve other persons for whom decision making responsibilities would be too overwhelming" (p. 166). One size does not fit all. What is important is that each person's preferences are first determined and then respected. Collaborative partnership is a complex approach to care, and many factors influence it. These factors will be fully discussed in Chapter 4.

Finally, in some of the studies just discussed it would probably be safe to assume that many of the respondents did not have the experience of working collaboratively with a professional and could only respond to questions about their involvement in their care based on the type of relationship they had experienced. In recent years, health care delivery has changed and some nurses have begun to work collaboratively with people. When researchers study people who have experienced a collaborative relationship with a professional, the study results begin to paint a somewhat different picture of people's desire to participate with professionals in their care.

WHAT DO PEOPLE WHO HAVE EXPERIENCED A COLLABORATIVE PARTNERSHIP SAY ABOUT THIS EXPERIENCE?

Interviews were conducted with families who had a family member living with chronic illness and who received care at the Family Nursing Unit at the University of Calgary (Robinson, 1996). Four of the five families interviewed expected to have a collaborative, nonhierarchical relationship with the nurse, whereas one family did not. This one family perceived the nurse to be the expert and expected the nurse to tell them how to deal with their situation. In their first contact with the nurse, the nurse used a collaborative approach and emphasized the family's strengths and abilities to deal with their situation. As a result, this family found that their view of how they wanted to work with the nurse changed. They quickly shifted their view in favor of looking for their own solutions and working collaboratively with the nurse.

In five different studies, done by five different teams of researchers in three different regions of Canada, families had very similar things to say about their experience working with a nurse who used a collaborative approach to care. The following paragraphs discuss sample comments made by different participants of these studies.

An experimental study was conducted to assess the effectiveness of a year-long collaborative nursing intervention, based on the McGill Model of Nursing, on the psychosocial adjustment of children living with a chronic illness (Pless et al., 1994). The intervention was effective in improving child adjustment, and parents whose child's adjustment had improved were interviewed to determine how those positive changes had come about. One parent explained, *"She [the nurse] was asking questions about it instead of telling us what to do."* Another parent stated, *"It was fun, because she [the nurse] didn't say, 'Well do this or that.' Instead the nurse would say, 'Think about it and you will tell me next time what you would like to do.' Then she would call back and I would tell her what I thought we should do"* (Ezer, Bray, & Gros, 1997, p. 375).

Families who had a family member living with a chronic illness and who received care at the Family Nursing Unit of the University of Calgary were asked to describe helpful nursing behaviours (Robinson, 1996). "It wasn't them [the nurses] telling us [what to do]. It was them helping us realize what we needed to do and then we did it together" (p. 165). People living with a chronic psychiatric illness were asked to describe how the nurse who utilized a collaborative approach worked with them (Moudarres, Fabijan, & Ezer, 2000). One participant noted: *"She [the nurse] let me be me. I got to talk about what I wanted to talk about, not what she thought I should. When I went to family therapy before, the therapist told me that I must have been sexually abused as a child on the first meeting. That is without even getting to know me. I never went back."*

The Comox Valley Nursing Centre in British Columbia (Attridge et al., 1996; Clarke & Mass, 1998) was a nursing project that incorporated a collaborative partnership approach in a primary care context. Clients described how the nurses helped them discover the "answers within themselves." They felt that their health concerns were heard by the nurse and understood, and that their care was being more effectively managed as a result (Attridge et al., 1996). Clients were asked what the nurse had done that was helpful, and the two most frequently mentioned helpful nursing behaviours were these: "Acting as though the client was responsible for directing their own health care" and "Ensuring that clients understood information and that choices were theirs to make" (p. 98). For example, one client stated, "They respected me totally and encouraged me to do what I wanted to do" (p. 99).

Chausse (2003) examined outpatient psychiatric patients' perceptions of their relationship with a nurse who used a collaborative partnership approach. One participant's comment summed up the thoughts of many. He noted, "Collaboration, it was what makes the difference in therapy" (p. 28). Participants were clearly able to distinguish the type of relationship they had with different nurses and other professionals, and were able to compare and contrast the outcomes of each type of relationship. They reported that they highly valued the collaborative partnership type of relationship.

For the participants of these studies, a key feature of their experience with collaboration was that the agenda for work and the pace and timing of the work were determined by them in discussion with the nurse, rather than by the nurse alone. Moreover, some people highlighted how the nurse helped them to change or achieve their goals by not telling them what to do. In essence, collaboration meant that the nurse helped them to help themselves. Although nurses have believed that a collaborative approach would help bring about people's desired change and growth, these studies indeed provide evidence that many families want this type of relationship with their health care provider and find that this type of approach can be particularly useful in bringing about change.

WHAT DO NURSES AND OTHER PROFESSIONALS SAY ABOUT COLLABORATION?

When most people consider the benefits of collaboration they tend to think of the benefits for people and not how this approach may benefit professionals in their practice. Lenrow and Burch (1981) have argued that when professionals approach their clients as collaborators "whose active contributions the professionals depend on in order to be able to use their own skills effectively" (p. 252), it benefits both the professional and the people with whom they work.

Studies of health professionals' (i.e., nurses, physician, psychologists, social workers, and occupational therapists) perceptions of people-professional partnerships have found that most believe that collaboration between professionals and patients is desirable (Jewell, 1994). Moreover, nurses perceive that joint efforts to work toward a common goal are the essence of collaboration and are important to helping people cope with different life situations (Paavilainen & Astedt-Kurki, 1997). Our nurse experts identified a number of benefits associated with a collaborative partnership approach.

When people are given the opportunity to be partners in their own care, they often enjoy this new role and feel satisfied with their care. Nurse Diane Lowden works with people living with multiple sclerosis and she explained, *"Some people are very motivated to enter into a collaborative relationship and are extremely receptive to the kind of questioning that involves them. They engage very readily and respond to this type of interaction. For other people this is a new idea that is a little bit foreign to them, and they're not really sure how to situate themselves in that sort of situation. They're used to medical encounters where they've had more direction and come to expect to have more direction. They're used to being told what to do."*

People develop greater competencies when they assume responsibility for dealing with their challenges and how these challenges are met. Nurse Cindy Dalton, who works with people living with chronic illnesses, explained, *"People own their success as well as the challenges of what it is that you're trying to work on with them. If you are working in partnership with them, they will take more initiative in trying to change things if it's not going well. They see that they have a role to play and that they are partners in shaping their care. They will own some of the success, and as a result gain competence."*

When people are active participants, they are more likely to apply what they have learned from one situation to the next. Nurse Jane Chambers-Evans, who practices in an intensive care setting, stated, *"I need to be careful not to take on the role of rescuer. There is a tendency, particularly in a situation of crisis, for nurses to try to solve all the problems. You're not going to gain anything by that. You just foster dependency and people are unable to move forward and do not gain anything from the experience. If people can't take some responsibility, then they may not learn the skills that they're going to need. It is a learning experience for the family to build on for the next time. If you haven't done that, then you haven't done your job very well."*

She went on to state, *"The rewards of a collaborative approach are great. You see persons and families better able to work with other health care professionals, particularly physicians, because you have done a lot of coaching and teaching, so they know how to be a partner. In working in partnership with the nurse, they have had the practice and they've experienced a different type of relationship. They now have a different model about how to relate to other health care professionals."*

CONCLUSION

Collaborative partnership has become an alternative approach to care, replacing the traditional hierarchical approach as the desired approach to care. The features of a collaborative partnership are (1) power sharing and sharing of expertise, (2) the pursuit of mutually agreed-on, person-centred goals, and (3) a dynamic process that requires the active participation and agreement of all partners in the relationship. Collaborative partnership involves continuously readjusting the relationship to achieve the right balance.

This approach to care has been embraced particularly by nursing because it fits well with nursing's core beliefs and values about how to care for people. It has gained acceptance due to a number of social, political, and professional forces, including consumerism and patient rights, primary health care and health promotion, the accessibility of health information, changes in thinking about nursing and ethical care, the shift from hospital-based to home-based care, and our current knowledge about how people change.

Much has been written about whether people want to collaborate with health care professionals. This is a rather simplistic way of thinking about collaborative partnership. A better way of thinking about collaborative relationships is to consider around what issues people want to collaborate, when they want to collaborate, and their style of collaboration. In the next few chapters we will describe the essential ingredients of collaborative partnership, the process and its phases, and the factors that will influence the degree to which collaborative partnership can be achieved.

KEY TERMS

collaborative partnership	person
cooperation	philosophical stance
participation	traditional hierarchical relationship

SUGGESTED READINGS

Allen, M. (1977). Comparative theories of the expanded role in nursing and its implications for nursing practice: A working paper. *Nursing Papers, 9,* 38-45. A seminal paper that identified the core concepts of the McGill Model of Nursing and distinguished it from a medical based model of nursing care.

Brearley, S. (1990). *Person participation: The literature.* London: Scutari Press. A comprehensive review of the literature on person participation and related concepts.

Cahill, J. (1998). Patient participation—A review of the literature. *Journal of Clinical Nursing, 7,* 119-128. Synthesizes the nursing literature on the concept of patient participation with particular emphasis on the forces that have given rise to partnership.

DeChillo, N., Koren, P. E., & Schultze, K. H. (1994). From paternalism to partnership: Family and professional collaboration in children's mental health. *American Journal of Orthopsychiatry, 64,* 564-576. This is an interesting research study on family and professional collaboration that examines the different aspects of collaboration and how it relates to person satisfaction with care.

Fromer, M. J. (1981). Paternalism in health care. *Nursing Outlook, 29,* 284-290. A discussion of the historical roots of paternalism in health care and why it is the dominant approach assumed by nurses.

Gallant, M. H., Beaulieu, M. C., & Carnevale, F. A. (2002). Partnership: An analysis of the concept within the nurse-client relationship. *Journal of Advanced Nursing, 40,* 149-157. A review of the literature on the concept of partnership between nurses and patients.

Greenfield, S., Kaplan, S. H., Ware, J. E., Martin Yano, E., & Frank, H. L. J. (1988). Persons' participation in medical care: Effects on blood sugar control and quality of life in diabetes. *Journal of General Internal Medicine, 3,* 448-457. An interesting study in which people with diabetes were taught how to collaborate in decision making with their doctor. Those who were able to collaborate had better blood sugar control.

Kirschbaum, M. S., & Knafl, K. A. (1996). Major themes in parent-provider relationships: A comparison of life-threatening and chronic illness experiences. *Journal of Family Nursing, 2,* 195-216. A rich description of parents' perception of how they work with health professionals to make decisions about their child's care.

McQueen, A. (2000). Nurse-patient relationships and partnership in hospital care. *Journal of Clinical Nursing, 9,* 723-731. A good overview of the background and forces that have led to collaborative approaches to nursing.

Pratto, F., & Walker, A. (2001). Dominance in disguise: Power, beneficence and exploitation in personal relationships. In A. Y. Lee-Chai & J. A. Bargh (Eds.), *The use and abuse of power: Multiple perspectives in the causes of corruption.* New York: Psychology Press. A fascinating discussion about how power-oriented individuals select careers in health care professions.

Stewart, M. J. (1990). From provider to partner: A conceptual framework for nursing education based on primary health care premises. *Advances in Nursing Science, 12,* 9-27. Summarizes the conceptual base that provides the rationale for a collaborative approach to nursing practice premised on primary health beliefs and assumptions but is applicable to other settings.

Sullivan, T. J. (1998). Consumers in health care, part II: Expert viewpoints. In T. J. Sullivan (Ed.), *Collaboration: A health care imperative* (pp. 561-590). New York: McGraw-Hill. Describes the rise of the consumer movement.

Young, L. E., & Hayes, V. E. (2002). *Transforming health promotion practice: Concepts, issues and applications*. Philadelphia: F. A. Davis. Describes health-promoting nursing practices in both health and illness situations through collaborative relationships between the nurse and the person from a Canadian perspective.

Chapter 2

THE ESSENTIAL INGREDIENTS OF A COLLABORATIVE PARTNERSHIP

When a family learns about a diagnosis, they may feel they've lost all power. In the process of working and collaborating with them, we want to bring forth the reality that they haven't lost all power.

—Nurse Jackie Townshend

After reading this chapter you should be able to:
- Identify the five essential ingredients of a collaborative partnership
- Describe the major characteristics of each ingredient
- Explain how each ingredient contributes to a collaborative partnership
- Describe the preconditions needed for power sharing

The five essential ingredients of a collaborative partnership are *sharing power, being open and respectful, being nonjudgmental and accepting, living with ambiguity,* and *being self-aware and reflective.* Although each of the ingredients of a collaborative partnership is discussed separately in this chapter, these ingredients are highly interrelated. A person's openness to the nurse is related to the nurse's acceptance of the person and his behaviour. Likewise, it will be difficult for a person to be open and share his thoughts and feelings with the nurse if he senses that the nurse is disapproving or judgmental of him. We examine each of these five ingredients in turn.

SHARING POWER

Sharing power is the heart of a collaborative partnership (Allen, 2000; Courtney, Ballard, Fauver, Gariota, & Holland, 1996; Henneman, Lee, & Cohen, 1995). How power is shared determines whether the nurse-person relationship will take on a more traditional hierarchical form (i.e., where the nurse is in the position of power) or whether the relationship will be more of a partnership in which power is shared. The way power is distributed is reflected in many functional aspects of the nurse-person relationship, such as how decisions are made or negotiated, whose opinion carries more weight, and who actually takes responsibility for the things that need to be accomplished (i.e., who does what) (Allen, 2000; Kirschbaum & Knafl, 1996).

During each phase of the nurse-person relationship, the distribution of power is evident. Power is evident in how decisions are made (i.e., who is involved in making decisions). The decisions that are made include what is going to be done (i.e., the agenda), who is responsible and accountable for carrying out the plan, and who is responsible for reevaluating the situation. Nurse Deborah Moudarres states, *"A collaborative partnership involves moving away from the nurse in the dominant role to a situation where the nurse is in a different type of role, such as that of a facilitator who has expertise in certain things. I think that clients are also experts, obviously, on where they've been, what they want to learn about, what they've already tried, and what's important to them. In a collaborative partnership we recognize that both partners have expertise."*

In the case of the traditional hierarchical nurse-patient relationship, the nurse is in charge, sets the agenda, and creates the plan of action, whereas the person's role is to comply with what the nurse decides. It thus follows that in a traditional hierarchical relationship the nurse also determines the effectiveness of the plan in achieving outcomes in terms of the nurse's criteria (Allen, 1977). Studies have shown that when patients have greater levels of involvement they are more likely to comply with their medical treatment regimen (Lahdenpera & Kyngas, 2001) and not feel powerless (Nordgren & Fridlund, 2001). When people are involved in making decisions about the plan of care, the plan is usually better suited to their needs.

A defining feature of a collaborative partnership is that power is shared. Power does not rest in the hands of one person. Within any given encounter power is fluid. The distribution of power is shaped by many factors, including the person and her situation, needs, preferences, abilities, physical condition, and mental well-being, as well as the nature of the situation. Thus, the distribution of power is ever changing. (Chapter 4 describes the factors that influence collaborative partnership.) At times, the nurse might assume more of the power and the person less power, whereas at other times the opposite might well be the case. At yet other times, both the nurse and the person share power more equally. Power sharing is not merely obtaining the person's perspective on her situation. True **power sharing** requires the participants to go beyond the exchange of perspectives to sharing in making decisions. This means that both partners set the agenda and determine a plan of action that best fits the person's realities. The work of implementing the plan is shared between the two partners based on their respective expertise, time, and energy. Although both partners participate in evaluating the outcomes, it is ultimately the person who decides whether the plan is working. It is her life and she has to live with the decisions.

The power structure within a collaborative partnership is egalitarian rather than hierarchical. As described in Chapter 1, in a hierarchical power structure, one person dominates over the other. In contrast, in an egalitarian power structure both partners are on the same level; each is learning from and being influenced by the other. Sharing power can be beneficial in and of itself, for both the person and the nurse. Jackie Townshend, who nurses families with children who have cystic fibrosis, explains: *"When a family comes to us and gets the diagnosis [of cystic fibrosis], they certainly feel that they don't want to be here. They may also feel that they've lost all power. Something has been taken away from them. In the process of working and collaborating with them, we want to bring forth the reality that they haven't lost all power. In fact, they can regain some of their power by learning about their child's illness, learning new ways of dealing with the illness, and developing new coping skills."*

Some studies suggest that some nurses have difficulty relinquishing and sharing power with people. A study of Australian nurses and patients from acute medical and surgical and extended care wards revealed that some nurses did not want to collaborate with patients. They wanted to make decisions for patients instead of helping them to make their own decisions (Henderson, 2003). These nurses thought that they "knew best" and that patients lacked medical knowledge. Observations of the nurses' behaviour further supported the idea that nurses used their power to maintain control of their patient and their care.

Nurses' ideas about power in nurse-person relationships are often embedded in their understanding of what it means to be professional. At the heart of this issue are nurses' notions about professional expertise and responsibility. The word *professional* comes from the word *profess* (Allen, 2000), which means "to know better." Some nurses think that to be a professional means to know better. Although nurses possess expert knowledge by virtue of their education and experience, so do people. The combined knowledge and experience of both the nurse and the person are essential for effective care. Being a professional means that the nurse is responsible and accountable for his nursing actions. However, this does not mean that the nurse has sole responsibility for achieving desired outcomes. Both the nurse and the person share responsibility for what happens.

Some nurses think that having a collaborative partnership means that the nurse never disagrees with the person and always follows her wishes. This is not so. First, the nurse's professional knowledge and expertise are important in a collaborative partnership relationship. The person has her own goals and the nurse too may have goals for the person. Typically, the nurse begins with the person's goals except in situations where safety is an issue; in such cases, the nurse's concern for the person's safety needs to take precedent. Even when the nurse begins to work with the person's goals, the nurse's goals may be placed on the back burner. When the timing is right, the nurse's goals may come to the fore.

Second, this idea that the person has all the power presupposes that there is a reverse hierarchy in a collaborative partnership. If this were the case, then the situation would be little different from that of a traditional hierarchical relationship. However, unlike the traditional hierarchical relationship, in which the health care professional holds most of the power, in this relationship the person would hold the power and therefore would, in effect, be functioning in a hierarchical way. This type of hierarchical relationship also has its problems because it ignores the nurse's professional knowledge, expertise, and the experience that accumulates through working with many people over time. A collaborative partnership is effective in part because the knowledge, expertise, and contributions of both partners are valued and tapped.

Consider this example from the practice of Gillian Taylor, a nurse who works with families who have children with rheumatoid arthritis: *"I think sometimes that the ideas about collaborative nursing can come across as being too 'pollyannaish.' Some people think that collaborating means that the nurse can never disagree with the patient and cannot voice her own opinion. A common situation that comes up often in my practice is that parents will minimize their child's symptoms for a time, skip appointments, and delay seeking care. Eventually, the child's disease really flares up, and the child is not getting treatment but needs to be. I've learned ways to respond so I can talk to parents about this. Paying no attention to what's happening feels schizophrenic to me. I can't ignore that the child isn't well and is limping. However, I'm certainly not going to say to the parents, 'Well why didn't you phone? I can't believe you waited so long to come.' But I may say, 'Things don't look as good as last time, and I'm actually a bit surprised that you didn't let us know. I bet there are good reasons; can we talk about them?' From a position of knowing these parents, I feel comfortable bringing my concerns up. I know that it might be better that they discuss this with me rather than with the physician who is going to say 'Aaah! Look at these knees. They are like cantaloupes! What's going on here?'"*

Collaborative partnership, in some situations, involves the nurse sharing a very different perspective with a client, challenging his view, or inviting him to see something differently. Again Nurse Gillian Taylor explains: *"Collaborative partnership is not just being nice. It is a process that allows you the space to ask sensitive or uncomfortable questions. Whenever you need to ask a question that may cause stress and worry, it is important to preface the question with a brief preamble so that the question is not misinterpreted or taken the wrong way. These approaches only serve to heighten collaborative partnership."*

Some people interpret the phrase *collaborative partnership* to mean that the decision-making power, responsibility, and workload are equally divided between the nurse and the person. When this is not the case, nurses sometimes think that they are not collaborating. In any partnership, one partner may assume more responsibility or play a more active role at any given time, and then responsibility may shift to the other partner at other points in time. The collaborative nature of a relationship often shifts over the course of one encounter or over the course of a relationship. In practice, depending on the circumstances, the nurse may assume more of the power, responsibility, or workload, whereas at other times the reverse may be the case. For example, in the immediate postoperative period, the nurse will assume greater responsibility for making decisions about the person's care. As the person recovers and feels able to take on more responsibility, the power for making decisions about care will shift to the person.

Knowledge Is Power

Knowledge and information are important determinants of power. The person who is thought to hold more knowledge and information tends to hold more of the power in the relationship. In a collaborative partnership, the nurse is aware of the knowledge and expertise she has and, at the same time, is also aware of the knowledge she does not have. In fact, in a collaborative partnership power is shared based on knowledge or expertise rather than on role or title (Henneman et al., 1995). Professionals are aware of the knowledge and expertise of the people they care for. A qualitative study of self-help groups (Banks, Crossman, Poel, & Stewart, 1997) found that patients valued the knowledge acquired through living with an illness, whereas health professionals' valued theoretical knowledge acquired through formal education.

In a collaborative partnership, both types of knowledge are recognized and valued by each partner. Each partner understands that it is the combination and sharing of their knowledge, skills, and expertise with each other that results in the best care. As a result of this recognition, in a collaborative partnership information and knowledge flow in both directions between partners. What distinguishes a collaborative partnership is not what knowledge each partner has, but rather how that knowledge is used and shared. Nurse Lucia Fabijan states, *"The nurse's knowledge is important. But the manner in which knowledge is shared is key. If you do it in a way that says 'I am the expert; I know precisely what's going on with you and what you need to do,' then you've lost some of what you might be able to achieve in creating a collaborative partnership with this family because they will not feel comfortable enough to be able to talk or express their ideas or be able to work toward whatever it is that they're going toward."*

Preconditions for Power Sharing

It all comes down to beliefs and attitudes. When these preconditions are not present, then power sharing is more difficult to achieve. First and foremost, both the nurse and the person need to believe in the importance and value of sharing power. The nurse and the person need to recognize that when they share power and work together as partners, they will be able to develop the best care for the person. Moreover, both partners need to believe that when the person participates in his care to the extent that the person desires, then the person is more likely to feel in control of his health care and be satisfied with it. In fact, a study of nursing based on a partnership model found that 89% of clients reported positive changes as a result of their work with a nurse (Attridge et al., 1996). Similarly, Krouse and Roberts (1989) found that people who actively negotiated decision making with the nurse experienced greater feelings of control over treatment decisions than people who were only partially involved and those who were not. This point is further elaborated in Chapter 4, where the factors that shape collaborative partnership are discussed.

The second precondition for successful power sharing is that each partner has to believe that he or she has something to contribute and something to gain from collaborating. Furthermore, each partner must also feel comfortable assuming some of the power by sharing in decision making and taking on responsibility for the care and what happens.

If the nurse sincerely believes in this approach and is committed to it, then she will always work with the ultimate goal of sharing power with the person and will always be looking for opportunities to help the person take on power. Power sharing will look different with different people. The degree of power sharing will vary from person to person because not everyone is initially ready to—or even interested in—sharing power with a health professional.

When nurses encounter people who are reluctant to share power, they need to carefully assess the reasons for this:

- Does the person not believe in the value of power sharing?
- Is this idea new to the person?
- Is the person frightened by the idea that the health professional may not have all the answers?
- Does the person feel that she does not have the knowledge or skills to share power with the nurse?

If the person does not appreciate the value and importance of power sharing, then it may be helpful for the nurse to explain the benefits of this approach. If the person feels that she has nothing to contribute, then the nurse needs to highlight and use the person's expertise, knowledge, and skill whenever possible. The nurse may also need to point out what the person has contributed and link this contribution to what has happened or has been achieved. How this can be accomplished is more fully described in Chapter 7, where our clinical experts address this challenge.

BEING OPEN AND RESPECTFUL

A collaborative partnership requires that each partner be open to the other and with each other. There are several aspects of openness. The most fundamental aspect of **openness** is a willingness to develop a relationship with the other person. Both partners must want to engage in a relationship. By virtue of their respective roles (i.e., health care provider and health care seeker), it seems that both partners would want to form a relationship with the other. However, in reality this is not always the case. Some nurses are reluctant to become involved with people and prefer that their interactions with other people be limited to the presenting medical concern. On the other hand, some people do not expect or want to form a relationship with the nurse. They view the nurse as someone who performs tasks, such as taking blood pressure and giving medications, and do not see any benefit from this type of involvement. Nurse Jane Chambers-Evans explains, *"There has to be an openness. First they have to be open to even enter into some kind of relationship with you. The second is that they need to feel that they're going to gain something from having a relationship with the nurse."*

A second aspect of openness is that both the nurse and the person must be willing to share information, ideas, and perspectives with one another and to hear what the other has to say (MacGillivary & Nelson, 1998). It is important that each partner be knowledgeable and have an understanding of the other's perspective. In initial encounters, openness means being curious and interested about the person's understanding of his situation, its meaning and importance, and being open to seeing the situation through the other person's eyes. A qualitative study of Swedish nurses' first encounters with parents of newborn children found that during the first encounter, the nurse's openness and receptiveness to the family's situation laid the foundation for a good reciprocal relationship (Jansson, Petersson, & Uden, 2001). The nurses stated that openness required them to "see" each family, listen carefully to them, allow the family to guide the conversation, and not dwell on information that was too medical or irrelevant to the family.

Nurses show openness through the questions they ask, how the questions are asked, how they listen to the responses to these, and then how they respond. In fact, Robinson (1996) reported in a study of families coping with chronic illness that the family appreciated when nurses listened carefully and asked relevant questions in response to what they had shared. As Nurse Margaret Eades explains, *"There needs to be openness in a collaborative partnership, and one aspect of that is to start where the person is. For me, I'm going to want to learn more about their issues and concerns and their readiness to work on them. I try to keep things open so they can explain what's important to them."*

Nurse Eades describes an example of considering the perspective of the other person from her practice with oncology patients and their families: *"There have been so many times when I have encountered a family who says to me, 'Just don't tell my mother that she has cancer. Couldn't we just give her some chemotherapy without her knowing?' I need to be open to understanding why they want this, what their fears are, and what their understanding of their mother is and her response to this situation. I am continually dancing to try to find ways to create a win-win situation out of this difficult situation."*

Nurse Chamber-Evans explains, *"If people have a feeling that you are coming with your agenda and that they are not going to have a part to play other than to listen and be told what to do, then the doors will close."*

A third aspect of openness involves a willingness to experiment, change, and learn something new. Nurses' best teachers are the people they are caring for. It is through these experiences coupled with their theoretical knowledge that nurses become experts (Schon, 1987). Nurse Irene Leboeuf describes a situation from her practice: *"The patient was a 36-year-old man, who was diagnosed with a malignant brain tumour. I had known him for more than a year, and we had been discussing the meaning of this event and how he could reframe this devastating experience to bring something positive into his life. I suggested that he write an article about his experience for our newsletter. The process of reflecting on this experience and telling his story brought him a sense of peace as he discovered his strengths. It was a useful exercise for him, but I learned so much about him and the meaning of his life from reading that story. He had surgery again yesterday, and I gave this article to the nurses taking care of him. By reading about him and what he had gone through, it gave these nurses a different perspective about the person they were nursing."*

Openness to change or learn is a fundamental requirement on the part of the person. The person has to want to change or learn and be ready for this. Nurse Joann Creager explains, *"There needs to be from the client or the family members some openness to learning, even if it's just a little glimmer of light. Some willingness to try something a little bit new is necessary to pursue health goals."*

Openness and respect go hand in hand. Respect requires openness and openness communicates respect. As Nurse Jane Chambers-Evans says: *"You cannot even begin a collaborative partnership if there is no respect for the person in front of you."*

Collaborative partnership requires each partner to value and respect the knowledge, skill, experience, and expertise that each partner brings to work together. Respect is necessary if people are going to actively participate in their health care (MacIntosh & McCormack, 2001). **Respect** for one another's roles and responsibilities is a critical feature of the collaborative nurse-person relationship (McCann & Baker, 2001). The nurse must see the person as a competent, capable partner who can, to varying degrees, participate in different ways in the partnership. Respect for one another's competencies is perceived as an important feature of partnership or of a collaborative approach (Attridge et al., 1996; Bidmead, Davis, & Day, 2002; Clarke & Mass, 1998; Coulter, 1999; Paavilainen & Astedt-Kurki, 1997). A study of people living with chronic illness (Thorne & Robinson, 1988) found that when people felt health professionals did not acknowledge and accept their competence in managing their illness, they became dissatisfied with their relationships with those professionals.

Respect also involves knowing that other people often have a perspective, an opinion, and ways of coping and solving problems that may differ from our own. Respect means honouring these differences and looking for common ground to manage these differences in ways that will best benefit the person.

Openness on the part of both partners is the key to successfully achieving a plan that fits. Without openness and a freedom to express what one feels, a common understanding, an appreciation of the other's position and perspective, and a mutually agreed-on plan cannot be achieved. Openness and respect lead to trust, and trust is fundamental to any relationship. But unlike a traditional hierarchical relationship in which the person needs to trust the nurse, in a collaborative partnership the person also needs to trust the nurse, but equally important is that the nurse needs to trust the person. Only then can the nurse and person enter into a collaborative partnership. The nurse needs to be able to trust the person's knowledge and abilities and willingness to work together.

BEING NONJUDGMENTAL AND ACCEPTING

A collaborative partnership requires that both partners be tolerant and nonjudgmental of the other. Being **nonjudgmental** means showing tolerance for another person's beliefs, values, behaviours, or perspectives. On the part of the nurses, it means that they are not critical or condemning of the person and her behaviour. Being nonjudgmental does not mean that nurses do not have their own set of beliefs, values, or opinions that may differ from those of the person. It does mean that they try to understand the person's perspective. As Nurse Deborah Moudarres describes: *"I find in psychiatry that the patients often come with a lot of feelings of shame and guilt because they feel that they've done something wrong or that they've pursued a kind of maladaptive way of coping or adjusting. It's very important right from the start—in terms of both engaging the person and developing a collaborative partnership—to have an accepting attitude."*

Nurse Jackie Townshend further explains: *"Being nonjudgmental doesn't mean that we don't have our own beliefs. It doesn't mean you're a blank slate. If a patient tells you about incest or something terrible, being nonjudgmental does not mean that these revelations do not have an impact on you and you don't feel 'My God, it's a horrible thing to have happened.' You do have your own beliefs, but that's not part of it. Being nonjudgmental means trying to understand where the client is coming from."*

The person also has to be open, nonjudgmental, and accepting of the nurse. Many people have preset ideas about the role of the nurse. They might not see the nurse as someone who can help them because the nurse is too young, too old, the wrong gender (e.g., male nurses), or lacks knowledge or experience. (See Chapter 7, in which one of the "Ask the Expert" questions provides a more detailed discussion of this issue.)

LIVING WITH AMBIGUITY

In a traditional hierarchical relationship, the nurse can often predict the course of events. In this type of relationship the nurse is in the "driver's seat." The nurse sets the agenda and makes the decisions about what to do. In a collaborative partnership, there are two "drivers." Thus, it is not always clear to either the nurse or to the person how the situation will unfold. The **ambiguity** in collaborative work requires that both the nurse and person be able to tolerate uncertainty and unpredictability for a period of time.

A collaborative partnership requires a shared understanding of the focus of work and the direction that the work takes. Thus, in a collaborative partnership the nurse may find that she needs to spend more time working with the person in defining the issues, setting the direction of the work, determining what will be accomplished, and so forth. Because the nurse is assisting the person to arrive at these decisions, this process takes time (Attridge et al., 1996). The nurse may often find herself in uncertain and unpredictable circumstances. Furthermore, many of the people that nurses collaborate with are coping with illness. The experience of living with illness involves dealing with many expected and unexpected events, which further contributes to the uncertainty and unpredictability of nursing in a collaborative way.

The person too needs to understand that collaborative problem solving requires time and patience. The person needs to be able to understand that there may be no "quick fixes" and be able to tolerate ambiguity. In the long run, the most effective plan emerges from a thorough understanding of the person's situation. To create this plan together, both partners have to gain a clearer, more precise understanding of the person's situation and then sort out what each brings to the situation and how best to work effectively together toward achieving their goals.

This is not to say that either the nurse or the person is passive, just waiting for things to happen, or that they do not plan for the future. Nurse Heather Hart, who works in palliative care, further elaborates on the importance of this ingredient: *"The nurse needs to be able to live in murky waters. There needs to be a willingness to take cues from the client and understand that everything is not going to proceed in a linear fashion. The nurse needs to learn how to be comfortable with situations that are not that clear. If the nurse is really going to engage with families, then you will be dealing with the give and take, and you have to take cues from them. They're going to determine the course as much as you are, maybe more—probably more—so you can't go in with a fixed idea of what the outcome is going to be. It takes a certain amount of flexibility and risk to nurse in this way because the direction may not be clear from the start."*

Given that much of the process of collaborative partnership involves being able to tolerate ambiguity or deal with unpredictability and uncertainty in situations that are themselves in a state of flux, it is essential for both the nurse and the person to be flexible and adaptable. Without some degree of flexibility, a working partnership will be difficult to maintain. Consequently, the relationship may cease to be collaborative and take on a more traditional hierarchical feel, or the relationship may deteriorate or even end.

BEING SELF-AWARE AND REFLECTIVE

Many processes take place within a collaborative partnership, including sharing one's thoughts and feelings, problem solving, negotiating, and decision making. All of these processes involve a delicate balance among the needs, agendas, goals, perspectives, and preferences of each partner. A successful balance in these areas will be more likely to occur if partners are able to understand themselves and each other and understand the situation from the other person's perspective. A successful partnership requires not only self-awareness, but also an awareness of the other person. This awareness should include the dynamics of what is going on within the relationship and the impact that one's own behaviour is having on the other. This involves a continuous monitoring of how the partners are working together.

Reflection is a mode of operation that helps professionals make sense of practice (Clarke, James, & Kelly, 1996). It is becoming a major technique for gaining self-awareness. Nurse Cindy Dalton elaborates on this idea: *"There really is a need for the nurse to have some level of self-awareness and to really reflect on what she says and does, and the impact that has on the person. The nurse needs to think about the content of what she's discussing and also how the process is unfolding. She needs to be able to step back when necessary and see that there is important information that the person needs to share."*

Reflection is a useful tool in any relationship, but is essential to a successful collaborative partnership. Reflection in a collaborative partnership relationship is useful for these reasons:

- It fosters an individualized and flexible approach to care. People's health situations are complex, multifaceted, and often require the development of a plan that is tailored or customized to the individual's needs (Schon, 1987).
- It enhances the visibility of therapeutic work and enables one to monitor the effectiveness of the work over time (Greenwood, 1998).
- It fosters the shifting and redistribution of control and power from one person to another through its mechanism of continuous monitoring.
- It fosters the recognition and management of negative feelings that might arise that can interfere with the relationship (McQueen, 2000).

In a collaborative partnership not only does the nurse engage in reflection, so does the person. **Reflection** can occur during the partners' interactions, but also after and between encounters (Greenwood, 1998). The use of reflection in practice is further discussed in Chapter 5 on nursing strategies. Box 2-1 provides a summary of the essential ingredients of a collaborative partnership.

Box 2-1	The Essential Ingredients of a Collaborative Partnership

- Sharing power
- Being open and respectful
- Being nonjudgmental and accepting
- Living with ambiguity
- Being self-aware and reflective

CONCLUSION

The essential ingredients of a collaborative partnership are sharing power, being open and respectful, being nonjudgmental and accepting, living with ambiguity, and being self-aware and reflective. Of these essential ingredients, the driver is sharing power. A collaborative partnership is all about the sharing of power and how power is distributed between the two partners. Power sharing does not mean that at all times in the relationship the power is equally distributed between partners. But it does mean that both partners have some degree of control, participate in decision making, and take responsibility for what is achieved in their work together. Sharing of power between partners can only occur when there is openness and respect within a nonjudgmental and accepting environment. It also has the best chance of occurring and being effective when each partner is able to "live in murky waters," develop a sense of self-awareness, and reflect on the situation and what is happening in their partnership.

KEY TERMS

ambiguity	**power sharing**
nonjudgmental	**reflection**
openness	**respect**

SUGGESTED READINGS

Attridge, C. B., Budgen, C., Hilton, A., McDavid, J., Molzahn, A., & Purkis, M. E. (1996). Report of the evaluation of the Comox Valley Nursing Centre. Victoria, BC: University of Victoria. Describes the evaluation of a demonstration nursing project based on a collaborative partnership approach to practice, and provides evidence that people value such a nursing approach. Makes recommendations about the implementation of this approach in practice.

Gallant, M. H., Beaulieu, M. C., & Carnevale, F. A. (2002). Partnership: An analysis of the concept within the nurse-client relationship. *Journal of Advanced Nursing, 40,* 149-157. A concept analysis of partnership based on a critical review of the literature.

Greenwood, J. (1998). The role of reflection in single and double loop learning. *Journal of Advanced Nursing, 27,* 1048-1053. Describes the purposes of reflection in professional practice.

Henneman, E. A., Lee, J. L., & Cohen, J. I. (1995). Collaboration: A concept analysis. *Journal of Advanced Nursing, 21,* 103-109. Describes the model, contrary, and related cases of using a collaborative or noncollaborative approach.

Kralik, D., Koch, T., & Wooton, K. (1997). *Journal of Advanced Nursing, 26,* 399-407. An interesting study of patients' perceptions of those nursing behaviours associated with nursing engagement.

McDowell, T. (2000). Practice evaluation as a collaborative process: A client's and a clinician's perceptions of helpful and unhelpful moments in a clinical interview. *Smith College Studies in Social Work, 70,* 375-387. An illustrative case study of a client–social worker interaction delineating the major features of a collaborative approach in practice.

Chapter 3

THE SPIRALLING MODEL OF COLLABORATIVE PARTNERSHIP

I engage people in exploring . . . what . . . they need and want, and how they want to do it. I explain that I am the expert at helping them to identify and explore their concerns and facilitate their problem solving, but . . . only they know what the situation means—and what may work best.

—Nurse Deborah Moudarres

After reading this chapter you should be able to:
- Identify the four phases of the collaborative partnership
- Describe the defining features of each phase of the collaborative partnership
- Describe the role of the nurse and the role of the person in each of these phases
- Explain four different scenarios that may occur after the reviewing phase of the collaborative partnership

---

Although the phases and processes within the nurse-person relationship have been well described, only a few have identified the phases within the nurse-person relationship premised on a collaborative approach (Bidmead, Davis, & Day, 2002; Courtney, Ballard, Fauver, Gariota, & Holland, 1996; Roberts & Krouse, 1988, 1990; Williamson, 1981). Recognizing the lack of empirically based study in this area, Moudarres and Ezer (1995) systematically examined the practice of community health nurses in a setting where nurses used the McGill Model of Nursing (Gottlieb & Rowat, 1997) as their framework of practice and identified the phases and processes involved in a collaborative partnership approach, which they have called the **Spiralling Model of Collaborative Partnership**. This chapter presents an overview of this model. Although developed from the practice of community-based nurses, the Spiralling Model of Collaborative Partnership has been validated with other populations such as

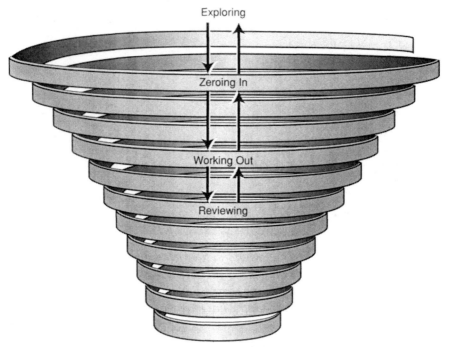

Figure 3-1 The four phases of collaboration. (Adapted from unpublished manuscript by Deborah Moudarres.)

psychiatric patients (Moudarres, Fabijan, & Ezer, 2000) and is applicable to any clinical population.

Within the Spiralling Model of Collaborative Partnership there are four inter-related phases: (1) exploring and getting to know each other, (2) zeroing in, (3) working out, and (4) reviewing (Figure 3-1). In each of these phases, the nurse and the person each have a distinct, yet reciprocal role to play. The term *spiralling model* derives from the nature of the process. Within any of the four phases the nurse and person can spiral forward to the next phase or spiral backward to any previous phase. Moreover, at each phase of the process the goal is to narrow the focus (without losing sight of the total picture of the person's situation) so that the work between the person and nurse proceeds from broad, general exploration to a more specific focus.

PHASE 1: EXPLORING AND GETTING TO KNOW EACH OTHER

The **exploring phase,** in which the partners to a collaborative relationship get to know each other, is the initial phase of the collaborative partnership process (Figure 3-2). Like any other relationship, the initial phase is characterised by

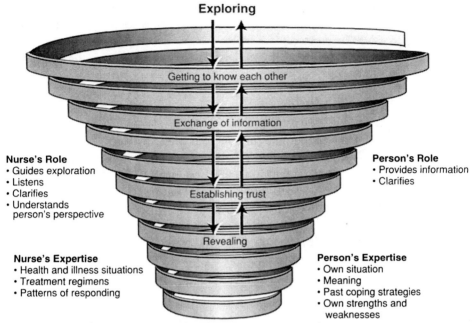

Exploring

Getting to know each other

Exchange of information

Nurse's Role
• Guides exploration
• Listens
• Clarifies
• Understands
  person's perspective

Establishing trust

Person's Role
• Provides information
• Clarifies

Revealing

Nurse's Expertise
• Health and illness situations
• Treatment regimens
• Patterns of responding

Person's Expertise
• Own situation
• Meaning
• Past coping strategies
• Own strengths and
  weaknesses

Figure 3-2   Exploring. (Adapted from unpublished manuscript by Deborah Moudarres.)

activities that enable each partner to become acquainted. This is accomplished through exchanging information, establishing trust, and revealing concerns.

Exchanging Information

The person's role at this point in phase 1 is to share information about his concerns. The initial information provided by the person may be concrete and factual. The nurse's role is twofold. First, she helps the person to share his concerns and to describe his experience. Second, the nurse provides information about her role and what she has to offer. It is crucial for the nurse to understand what the particular concern means to *this* person. As the nurse and the person explore the situation in a more comprehensive way, the nurse is not only listening for the "facts" but is also listening to understand the importance and significance of the issue to the person and his family. For the nurse to be able to listen to the person and begin to perceive the situation through his eyes, the nurse must be open and responsive. This requires the nurse to have some level of self-knowledge and be aware of her own beliefs about the problem or issue. (See Chapter 2 on ingredients and Chapter 4 on the factors that affect a collaborative partnership.) The nurse's responsibility is to gather as much information as the person is willing to divulge through sensitive, open-ended questioning, active listening, and observing of nonverbal behaviour.

Sensitivity refers to the nurse's being able to read and respond to the person's cues about what topics he is willing to share, when he is ready to discuss an issue, and how much he is willing and ready to divulge.

The nurse may use the following types of questions to explore the nature and meaning of the concern:

- Tell me about this concern.
- How long has this been of concern?
- What effect is this concern having on your life?
- What other issues are related to it?
- What have you done to deal with this concern? What happened? Was it effective? If so, how did you know it was effective?
- Who helps you deal with this concern?
- What do you think your positive characteristics are? What can you do well? How might that help you in this situation?
- What would you like to see happen?
- If you could imagine that things were better, what would such a situation look like?

The nurse's success in connecting with the person is based not only on the questions that are asked, but more importantly on the way in which the questions are posed, the timing of these questions within the overall relationship and the encounter, and how the nurse reacts to what the person reveals. The nurse's ability to be nonjudgmental, accepting, and interested in the person and not just the "illness" is critical at this point in the relationship-building process.

The expertise of both the person and the nurse is brought to bear in this phase of information exchange. The nurse possesses "expert" knowledge about health and illness situations, medical and nursing treatment regimens, and people's patterns of responses to and coping with health and illness situations. Although the nurse may have expert knowledge about health situations, ultimately she recognizes that the person knows his own situation best.

Many assume that because the nurse and person are partners, each can fill the other's shoes within the relationship. In fact, at this phase and throughout the process, partnerships work best when there is a clear understanding of one's own role and the role of the other. When each partner has a clear understanding of his or her own role and what to expect from the other partner, then the stage is set for a well-functioning partnership.

Establishing Trust

The first few encounters are important inasmuch as they set the tone for working collaboratively within the partnership (Jansson, Petersson, & Uden, 2001). To get the person to be an active partner in the relationship and to develop trust in the nurse, it is important that the nurse begin with what is of importance or of uppermost concern to the person. The nurse recognizes that it is the person's perceptions and how the person has constructed meaning of the events that affects how the person feels and behaves. Thus, when the nurse actively seeks and values the person's opinion or perspective, then the nurse communicates to the person her respect for him, and that it is his concerns and points of view that will be the focus of care. Moreover, this approach also conveys that the person can freely express his opinion or perspective without being judged.

During these first encounters, people often have very concrete requests for help (e.g., "What should I be feeding my newborn baby?"). In nursing practice, this request is often presented in the form of a question or concern about the person's medical condition. People may initially present this type of request because they know that nurses possess knowledge and expertise about medical conditions and their treatment. However, they may not be aware that nurses also have the knowledge and expertise to deal with a broader range of individual and family concerns. These initial concrete requests may also serve as the person's "test" of the nurse's competency and responsiveness, and they may facilitate the development of trust. How the nurse responds to these initial concerns will affect whether the person develops trust in the nurse, returns for subsequent encounters, or sees the nurse as an important resource who can help the person deal with other health-related concerns.

During this phase of collaborative partnership, the nurse's primary role is to understand the person's situation, whereas the person's primary role is to help the nurse understand her concerns. While the person is doing most of the talking and the nurse is probing, the person may also be "testing" to decide whether she has confidence in the nurse's abilities. Testing comes in a variety of forms. For example, one common way in which a person may test a nurse is by asking the nurse about something that she already knows a lot about. A patient who is knowledgeable about a medication may ask the nurse about the side effects, even though she herself is well versed in the subject. The patient does this to assess the nurse's knowledge and competency. Only if the nurse passes this test will the person invest in the relationship.

People may also test the nurse's willingness to work collaboratively with them. A young couple asked one of our former graduate students what the recommended sleep position was for their newborn infant. They told the student that they had been placing their infant in the prone, or facedown, position. The student explained that the recommended position, based on the research evidence on sudden infant death syndrome, was to place infants on their backs for sleep. The student offered to give the parents more information about this, but also explained that it was up to the parents to decide what might be best for their child. At the next visit, the couple told the student that several health professionals had become annoyed with them on learning that they had been positioning their infant in the prone position. As a result, the couple decided not to continue seeing these other health care providers. Because of the student's approach, the couple wanted to continue working with the student on other parenting issues. Several weeks later, the couple had read the material on sleep position that the nurse had given them and decided to place their infant in the supine position.

Just as the nurse is getting to know who the person is, the person is also getting to know the nurse and what the nurse has to offer. When the nurse is genuinely interested in the person, is emotionally and physically present and available to them, and demonstrates that he is knowledgeable and competent, the person then begins to develop trust in the nurse. As the relationship evolves, each partner begins to trust the other. When this happens, the quality of the information that the person is willing to share often moves from superficial issues to issues of a more personal and sensitive nature.

Revealing Concerns

Once the person has established some level of confidence and trust in the nurse, and the nurse has developed some trust in the person, then the person may be ready to reveal or to deal with concerns of a more intimate, deeper nature. The nurse's role is to guide the person in examining her beliefs about the concern and to listen carefully to the person's story for clues that might reveal the underlying meaning of that concern. It can take time for the nurse and person to "peel back" and understand the deeper meaning or significance of the true nature of the person's concerns. For example, Mrs. Tucci came to see the nurse because she had headaches that caused her to miss work for several days. Her anxiety about these headaches persisted even after she and the nurse had devised an effective plan to manage the pain. On further exploration the nurse discovered that Mrs. Tucci's mother had died suddenly from an aneurysm when Mrs. Tucci was a teenager—that is, the nurse discovered that the true meaning of Mrs. Tucci's headaches went far beyond her concern for her work absences.

The exploring phase is one that the nurse and person may revisit or "spiral" back to at any time in the process. Although there may still be things to discover about the person and her concerns, or about the situation, at some point both the nurse and the person may feel they have sufficient information to move on to the next phase of zeroing in. Note that in some situations the nurse and person might never move on from this first phase.

Some nurses believe that collaborative partnership just involves the nurse asking the person about his perspective on the situation and the nurse taking this perspective into consideration when devising the plan of care. However, this is just a first step in the process of working collaboratively—it is not yet a true collaborative partnership. The person has to be a partner in decision making, not just a consultant.

PHASE 2: ZEROING IN

The **zeroing-in phase** is characterised by efforts to identify specific, workable goals and to prioritize these goals (Figure 3-3).

Clarifying Goals

Some people clearly know what they want and where they would like to go. Other people have difficulty articulating what they would like to achieve (i.e., their goals), and still others may be able to articulate their goals but may do so in ways that are too vague (e.g., "I want to feel better") or too general (e.g., "I want to feel less anxious") to be workable. For those people who have difficulty articulating their goals or whose goals are too vague or too general, the focus of work in this phase of the spiralling model is to clarify goals. The greater the clarity and specificity of the goal, the easier it is for the nurse and person to develop a plan of action.

In the process of clarifying the person's goal, the nurse's primary role is to structure a discussion so that both the nurse and the person will come to more fully understand what the person wants to achieve. This technique of structuring a discussion is further described in Chapter 5. The nurse employs a variety of

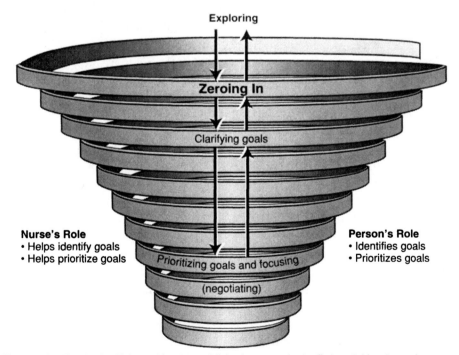

Figure 3-3   Zeroing in. (Adapted from unpublished manuscript by Deborah Moudarres.)

strategies to help the person articulate and clarify her goals, such as observing, active listening, posing purposeful questions, interpreting, validating, and rephrasing. At this point in the relationship, the nurse might also share with the person her ideas or impressions about the person's goal (i.e., the feasibility, the appropriateness of the timing, how the goal relates to the person's overall situation, or other things that need to be put in place before the person can enact the goal). The person's primary role at this time is to provide greater specificity in the identification of a particular goal.

If a person is unable to identify and describe his goals, does that mean a collaborative relationship will not work? Collaboration is based on the nurse's understanding of the person's goals and helping him to achieve those goals. Sometimes it may appear that the person has no goals, but the fact is that all people have goals. Humans are by nature goal directed. However, some people may have difficulty identifying or describing to others what they want to achieve. In some situations, the nurse needs to help the person understand what a goal is. The nurse can sometimes identify the person's goals by observing his behaviour, listening to what he would like to see happen, or asking him questions about what he is trying to achieve in a way that the person can relate to and understand. The nurse may need to explain that the person's behaviour is a reflection of something he is trying to achieve (i.e., a goal). What is important here is that the nurse helps the person label his behaviour and link it to a goal, thus linking behaviour with intention. In essence the nurse makes explicit what until now has been covert. At other times, the nurse may have to help people fine-tune their goals by helping them identify goals that are meaningful, realistic, and achievable.

Once the nurse and person are clear as to what the goals are, they are ready to move to the next step. In situations where there are a number of goals, the nurse and the person need to prioritize the goals and then focus on the top-priority goal. If the nurse and person are having difficulty clarifying the goal, it may be because they have zeroed in on a goal prematurely. In these cases, it may be necessary to spiral back to the first phase of exploring and getting to know each other to more fully understand the nature of the situation or their concerns.

Prioritizing Goals and Focusing

Prioritizing goals and focusing on a goal takes place through a process of negotiation. Negotiating may be required when the nurse and person have different goals, when they perceive the concerns somewhat differently, or when there are many goals that need to be prioritized. What is critical here is that both partners must be involved in negotiating if it is to be a truly collaborative effort. The nurse and the person assess what goals are of greatest importance, most amenable to change, or most likely to be resolved in a relatively reasonable period of time. The partners share their opinions with each other. **Negotiation** skills involve listening carefully to understand how the other partner is viewing the situation, being aware of and being able to communicate how one sees the situation, and explaining a viewpoint in ways that the other person can understand and appreciate. It also requires the skills of knowing how to find common ground, knowing whose perspective should be given greater weight, and knowing when and how to compromise. It is through the exchanging of ideas and weighing of costs and benefits that priorities are jointly chosen. Once the person and nurse have decided which concern or goal to focus on, they are ready to move into phase 3, the working-out phase.

PHASE 3: WORKING OUT

The **working-out phase** is the problem-solving phase of the collaborative partnership relationship (Figure 3-4). Two activities are involved in this phase: (1) considering alternatives and (2) trying out a plan. Once the nurse and person have zeroed in on what they want to work on, they are then ready to begin the actual work. The nurse's role at this time is to systematically guide and/or support the person's efforts through the identification of possible ways of dealing with the concern or reaching the goal(s).

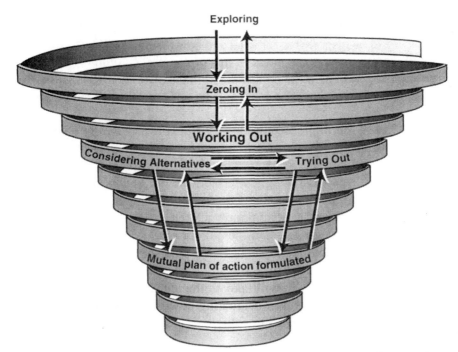

Figure 3-4   Working out. (Adapted from unpublished manuscript by Deborah Moudarres.)

Considering Alternatives

One method of generating alternative ways of achieving goals is through brainstorming (see Chapter 5). The nurse and the person, either together or alone, try to come up with as many ways of achieving the goal as they can think of so that they have many possible alternatives from which to choose. This phase requires that both the nurse and the person be open to ideas, flexible in their thinking, and willing to consider new ideas and approaches. The nurse may ask thought-provoking questions that might help generate options. The nurse may also inquire about what has been tried in the past and what has worked. Once a number of alternatives have been identified, then the next step is to evaluate the feasibility of each. Ultimately, the decision as to which option to try rests with the person.

Sometimes the person may have difficulty considering alternative ways of dealing with a concern or achieving a goal. When the person negates every suggestion or has difficulty brainstorming, then this may indicate that the concern has not been fully explored nor understood by either the person, the nurse, or both. The best way to proceed if this happens is to spiral back to the exploring or zeroing-in phases.

Trying Out a Plan

Once the person and the nurse have chosen an alternative, they are ready to decide who will be responsible for what and how the plan will be implemented. One of the major roles of the nurse in this phase of the collaborative partnership relationship is to help the person determine a plan of action that best suits him. The nurse then reviews the goals and the options selected and outlines the next steps.

In some cases, the implementation of the plan rests entirely with the person. The nurse's role may be only to support, coach, or serve as a model for the person during this period. A simple telephone call by the nurse may be enough to provide support designed to increase the successful implementation of the plan. In other cases, the major work of carrying out the plan may fall to the nurse because the person may lack the energy, motivation, skill, or confidence to do so, such as when the person is too ill or depressed. Note, however, that when the nurse implements the plan she does so with the intention that at some point in the future or in other situations (when the person is ready), it is the person who will take on the major work for implementing the plan. An important aspect of evaluating how well the plan is working is setting aside time for reviewing, which is phase 4 of the collaborative partnership.

PHASE 4: REVIEWING

The nurse and person need to review how well their plan is working or has worked (Figure 3-5). This entails setting aside specific time to deliberately review what has happened. The **reviewing phase** is an important phase of the Spiralling Model of Collaborative Partnership. It enables the person to understand what may be helping in bringing about change or what has allowed the person to achieve her goals. The process of reviewing makes what the person has learned from the experience more transparent to herself. When the person has greater insight and understanding as to why things happened and how they came about, she is more likely to apply this knowledge to future situations. Reviewing involves examining the alternatives that were implemented, how well the plan worked for the person and her situation, and whether the plan was effective. Although the nurse may voice her evaluation as to the success of a particular alternative action, it is the person who decides whether or not a goal has been satisfactorily met.

Moudarres, Ezer, and Schein (1997) described four possible scenarios resulting from the review phase:

1. The person no longer needs nursing care. If the presenting concern is resolved, the person and nurse may find that there are no other pressing

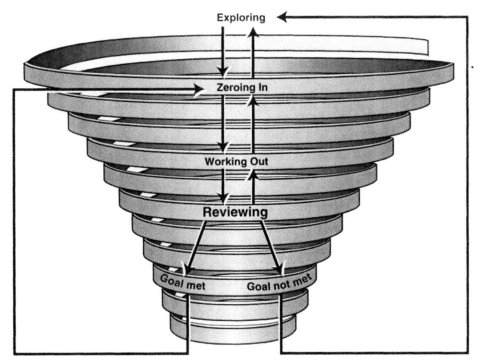

Figure 3-5   Reviewing. (Adapted from unpublished manuscript by Deborah Moudarres.)

concerns or goals. In some situations there may be additional concerns; however, the person may have the knowledge and skill or other resources to deal with these issues without further involvement of the nurse.

2. The initial concern has been met, but other concerns or a different or deeper meaning has been revealed. In this case, the nurse and person may spiral back to the zeroing-in phase. When the nurse helps the person deal successfully with her initial concerns, the person gains trust and confidence in the nurse and may become more open to dealing with other issues. For example, Mrs. Martinez was a very depressed and anxious postpartum mother who initially asked Nurse Moudarres to help her with some difficulties in breast-feeding. Mrs. Martinez attributed her anxiety and sadness to her inexperience with breast-feeding. However, after Mrs. Martinez and Nurse Moudarres explored her situation—that is, zeroed in on it—and dealt with the concerns about breast-feeding, when they reviewed what had transpired they found that although the breast-feeding concerns had been addressed Mrs. Martinez was still very sad and anxious. Nurse Moudarres, through gentle probing, discovered that Mrs. Martinez's sadness was related to the emergency hysterectomy she had immediately following the birth of her child. Even though Nurse Moudarres had been aware of this event, during their initial encounters Mrs. Martinez's verbal and nonverbal cues indicated to Nurse Moudarres that she was not yet ready to discuss her hysterectomy. Once Nurse Moudarres had gained Mrs. Martinez's confidence and trust by helping her successfully breast-feed, then Mrs. Martinez was open to discussing her feelings of loss and sadness related to her hysterectomy.

3. The initial goal was not achieved. In this case, the nurse and person may spiral back to the exploring and getting to know each other phase to reevaluate the issues and determine how best to proceed. Mr. Taylor was a 35-year-old man with bipolar disorder recently separated from his girlfriend (Moudarres et al., 2000). During the zeroing-in phase Nurse Fabijan and Mr. Taylor identified that Mr. Taylor's goal was to find low-cost housing. However, when Nurse Fabijan and Mr. Taylor reached the reviewing phase, Mr. Taylor had not yet applied for low-cost housing per the agreed-on plan. Although the nurse thought that the client was being avoidant, she kept these thoughts to herself. After some time, with little progress being made toward the identified goal, the nurse and Mr. Taylor spiralled back to the exploring phase to reassess whether this was in effect what Mr. Taylor really wanted to achieve. As they discussed the goal, Mr. Taylor revealed that a move to low-cost housing meant he would distance himself from his social network. Once Mr. Taylor had expressed his fears, he and Nurse Fabijan were able to zero in again, but now they worked to deal with Mr. Taylor's fears while not losing sight of his long-term goal. Within a year, Mr. Taylor applied for and moved into low-cost housing.

4. The nurse or the person, on reviewing their work together, decide that the person's needs would be better met by another nurse or health care professional. At this point, the nurse may refer the person to another professional.

CONCLUSION

Although many have identified the phases within the nurse-person relationship, none have clearly outlined the collaborative work that goes on within each of the phases of that relationship. The Spiralling Model of Collaborative Partnership provides nurses with a framework for collaborating with individuals and families. In conclusion, this process has a number of important features that warrant highlighting.

First, in a collaborative relationship, each partner has a distinct role to play at each phase in the model. Moreover, these roles are reciprocal and most often complementary. For example, in the exploring and getting to know each other phase, the nurse's role is to help the person identify and describe his concerns, whereas the person's role is to identify and describe to the nurse what is of concern to him.

Second, a key feature of the spiralling model is the fluid nature of the model and its phases. It is important to keep in mind that each phase of the process can occur almost simultaneously, which cannot be easily captured in a written description of this process. For example, in one encounter the nurse and person could be reviewing their progress on one concern, while at the same time exploring a related issue. Moreover, the process may not take place in a linear or in an invariant order. That is to say, the nurse and person could at any time proceed to the next phase, move ahead two phases, or spiral back to a previous phase. The way in which the nurse and person proceed depends on the nurse being responsive to what the person needs and what the situation requires at any given point in time.

KEY TERMS

exploring phase	**Spiralling Model of Collaborative Partnership**
negotiation	**working-out phase**
reviewing phase	**zeroing-in phase**

SUGGESTED READINGS

Egan, G. (2002). *The skilled helper: A problem-management and opportunity-development approach to helping* (7th ed.) Pacific Grove, CA: Brooks/Cole Publisher.

Ezer, H., Bray, C., & Gros, C. P. (1997). Families' description of the nursing intervention in a randomized control trial (pp. 371-376). In L. N. Gottlieb &

H. Ezer (Eds.), *A perspective on health, family, learning, and collaborative nursing: A collection of writings on the McGill Model of Nursing*. Montreal: McGill University School of Nursing. Families describe nursing behaviours that they view as helpful.

Gottlieb, L. N. (1997). Health promoters: Two contrasting styles in community nursing. In L. N. Gottlieb & H. Ezer (Eds.), *A perspective on health, family, learning, and collaborative nursing: A collection of writings on the McGill Model of Nursing* (pp. 98-109). Montreal: McGill University School of Nursing. Describes the roles that nurses can assume in helping people work towards their health goals.

Karhila, P., Kettunen, T., Poskiparta, M., & Liimatainen, L. (2003). Negotiation in Type 2 diabetes counseling: From problem recognition to mutual acceptance during lifestyle counseling. *Qualitative Health Research, 13,* 1205-1225. Describes the process of negotiation and its characteristics in actual nurse-person interactions.

McNaughton, D. B. (2000). A synthesis of qualitative home visiting research. *Public Health Nursing, 17,* 405-414. This systematic review of the literature on the home visiting practices of public health nurses revealed that building and preserving the relationship with the client is the central focus of home visiting. Describes the phases in the relationship and the roles of the nurse and client.

Morse, J. M. (1991). Negotiating commitment and involvement in the nurse-patient relationship. *Journal of Advanced Nursing, 16,* 455-468. Describes different types of mutual nurse-person relationships.

Morse, J. M., Deluca Havens, G. A., & Wilson, S. (1997). The comforting interaction: Developing a model of the nurse-patient relationship. *Scholarly Inquiry for Nursing Practice, 11,* 321-343. Distinguishes between interactions (encounters) and a relationship and the connection between interactions and relationships.

Robinson, C. A. (1996). Health care relationships revisited. *Family Systems Medicine, 16(1-2),* 7-25. Families describe what nursing behaviours are helpful.

Chapter 4

FACTORS THAT SHAPE THE
COLLABORATIVE PARTNERSHIP

*No single factor alone influences the collaborative partnership. With an
understanding of the factors that may influence the collaborative partnership,
the nurse can then purposefully work to create the conditions that will
maximize the person's active participation in this relationship.*
— Laurie N. Gottlieb and Nancy Feeley

After reading this chapter you should be able to:
- Have a greater appreciation of personal and situational factors and the
  roles they play in the collaborative partnership process
- Describe how nurse and person personal characteristics influence a col-
  laborative partnership
- Describe how nurse-person relationship factors influence a collaborative
  partnership
- Describe how environmental, organizational, or other situational factors
  influence a collaborative partnership
- Explain what the role of time and timing is in a collaborative partnership
- Use the assessment guide to help maximize the conditions that foster col-
  laborative partnership

Because the nurse assumes the leading role in initiating, developing, and setting
the tone of the collaborative partnership, the nurse needs to be aware of the
many, often varied factors that can influence the collaborative partnership and
its process. Dalton (2001) first developed the **Collaborative Partnership
Factors Assessment Guide.** This assessment guide outlines the factors that
influence the degree to which the nurse will be able to implement a collaborative partnership approach with the person and the degree to which the person
will partner with the nurse. In this chapter we have identified additional
factors, resulting in four major categories: (1) nurse factors; (2) person factors;

(3) relationship factors; and (4) environmental, organizational, and situational factors. This chapter describes this assessment guide beginning with the nurse and person factors and moving out to the wider environmental context in which the nurse-person relationship is situated.

The Collaborative Partnership Factors Assessment Guide can be used to assess the degree of collaborative partnership that can be expected within a particular nurse-person encounter. It also provides a guide for the nurse regarding how to develop and maintain a collaborative partnership. Nurse, person, relationship, and environmental factors need to be considered together, as no single factor alone influences the collaborative partnership.

Figure 4-1 shows how the various factors influence the collaborative partnership. It depicts a seesaw on which the nurse and person sit. The nurse and person are working together on the person's concerns and their mutually agreed-on goals (i.e., the agenda). The seesaw figure depicts the delicate balance of power that is

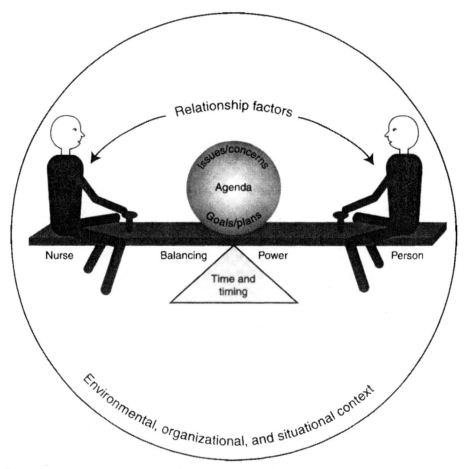

Figure 4-1 The factors influencing a collaborative partnership. (Adapted from Dalton, C. [2001]. Conditions for collaboration framework. Unpublished manuscript. Montreal, Quebec. McGill University School of Nursing.)

continually distributed and redistributed within the collaborative partnership or within any given encounter. The incline of the bench of the seesaw reflects the distribution or balance of power between the two partners. The balance of power is a function of each partner's personal characteristics, their situational circumstances, and the nature of their relationship and the environment in which the relationship develops. The balance of power is also a function of the person's needs, expectations, and preferences for how he wishes to work with the nurse. Ideally the nurse should always be working toward creating conditions that tip the balance of power in favour of the person having equal or greater power. Nurse Cindy Dalton explains how this operates in practice: *"Initially you may be less directive with somebody who can effectively problem solve, but be more directive with someone who has the expectation that the clinician should solve his or her problems (begin with the person's preference). Nonetheless, with somebody like that, over time you can be less directive as the person becomes more skilled or more comfortable with problem solving and assumes greater responsibility for the direction of his or her care. But you have to work with their abilities at that moment and shape the collaborative process over time."*

TIMING: KNOWING WHEN THE TIME IS RIGHT

We cannot underestimate the importance of time and timing in the development of a successful collaborative partnership. Time and timing is the fulcrum in Figure 4-1. By timing we are referring to how well the nurse is "in sync" with or "in tune" with the person and his needs *at any given moment*. The nurse needs to assess whether the time is right to maximize the conditions for collaborative partnership (Dalton, 2001). For example, if the person is acutely ill, he may not feel well enough to assume decision-making responsibilities with the nurse, and the time may not be right to maximize the conditions for collaborative partnership and shift the balance of power to him. Looking again at Figure 4-1, the incline of the bench of the seesaw in this example would be tipped in favour of the nurse having greater power at that particular point in the relationship. This shift is appropriate in this situation and reflects the nurse's responsiveness to the person's needs at that time. The nurse should constantly ascertain the degree to which the person wishes to be involved at any time, respect the person's preferred level of collaborative partnership, and adjust the form of collaborative partnership accordingly.

NURSE AND PERSON PERSONAL FACTORS

The personal characteristics and qualities of both the nurse and the person are major determinants of collaborative partnership. Given that the types of factors that influence the nurse and the person are similar, we discuss the nurse and person factors together. For example, the beliefs of both the nurse and the person are very important in influencing the collaborative partnership. However, the specific type of beliefs that the nurse holds may be very different than those that the person holds. The nurse and the person factors that affect the degree of collaborative partnership are as follows:

- Beliefs and expectations about the self, the other, and the relationship
- Knowledge of self and the health care situation or experience
- Critical thinking skills
- Learning styles
- Readiness
- Communication and interpersonal skills
- Physical and mental status

Beliefs and Expectations

Beliefs are the lenses through which we see the world. They affect what we attend to and how we behave. Beliefs shape our expectations, and both beliefs and expectations in turn shape the nature and form that the collaborative partnership takes.

Lenrow and Burch (1981) argued that beliefs about the "helping" and "helpee" roles are deeply embedded in our culture, and these beliefs make it difficult for both the professional and the person to perceive that the person can act as a partner with a helping professional. Professional training and education and the bureaucratic organization of hospitals and other health care institutions often reinforce these beliefs. Thus, a very important determinant of whether the nurse and person become collaborative partners is what the partners believe their own role should be and what they believe the role of the other person should be. DeChillo's study (1993) of the factors that influenced whether collaborative partnership took place between social workers and their clients revealed that the social workers' beliefs about client involvement in their care was the most influential factor in determining the nature of the relationship. Similarly, in a British study on parents' involvement in the care of their sick child, involvement was related to the health care professionals' expectations for parental involvement (Kirk, 2001). If the nurse believes people seeking care should be "seen and not heard," the nurse is more likely to adopt a traditional hierarchical approach in which the nurse expects the person she is caring for to follow her advice.

On the other hand, if the nurse believes that people have expertise and knowledge and that goals can best be achieved by actively involving people in their own care, then the nurse is more likely to adopt a collaborative partnership approach. A study of Canadian nurses and palliative care patients by Botoroff and colleagues (2000) found that there were four patterns of how nurses engaged patients in making choices about their care. These patterns ranged from "Opening up possibilities for the patient to choose" (i.e., the nurse respected the patient's agenda and assumed low control over the patient's choice) to "Offering pseudo choices" (i.e., offering the patient choices that were not real choices and assuming high control). Any particular nurse's use of one approach or another depended on the nurse's beliefs and values about giving patients the right to make choices in their care. In addition, if the person believes that health professionals are the experts who "know best" and whose role it is to take care of them, then they are less likely to want to function as a partner.

Knowledge

To work collaboratively, the nurse requires both clinical knowledge and knowledge of the situation. Clinical knowledge refers to both theoretical and experiential knowledge of people and families and how they respond and cope during periods of health, vulnerability, and illness. Every area of practice has specialized clinical knowledge. For example, in critical care nursing, some of the knowledge that nurses need to possess includes knowledge of the diagnosis and management of life-sustaining, physiological functions in unstable patients; the skilled know-how of managing a crisis; comfort measures for the critically ill; and communicating and negotiating multiple perspectives (Benner, Hooper-Kyriakidis, & Stannard, 1999). The nurse must also possess knowledge of the situation. This knowledge derives from getting to know the person and begins in the first phase of the collaborative partnership process and continues throughout the relationship (see Chapter 3).

The amount of knowledge that the person has may have an impact on her ability to collaborate (Kim, 1983). A descriptive study of hospitalized surgical patients' perceptions of factors that determined their participation in their own care decisions showed that how much they knew about a given issue determined how involved they felt they should be in these care decisions (Biley, 1992). For example, patients thought they should play a more passive role when technical care issues were involved, but preferred playing a major role in decisions that involved their activities of daily living while in hospital.

The person's own knowledge of the situation and what has been helpful in the past is also important in shaping the collaborative partnership. One of the person's primary roles in the collaborative process is for the person to share her unique understanding with the nurse (see Chapter 3). The person's knowledge of the situation and the degree to which she is willing to share this information is a key source of the person's power. In fact, the person might judge the nurse's competence and knowledge in light of her own expert knowledge that she has acquired in dealing with her own illness or that of a family member. Kirk (2001) found that parents who had in-depth knowledge of their own child and their child's complex health care needs used this knowledge to judge a professional's level of competence.

Critical Thinking Skills

The old adage "two heads are better than one" is very appropriate in the context of the collaborative partnership. Critical thinking skills involve assessing different pieces of information gathered at different times and then putting these pieces together to arrive at some understanding of the person's situation. It also involves linking past events to current situations. The combined analytical abilities or critical thinking skills of the person and the nurse make it more likely that effective ways of achieving goals will be found.

Critical thinking skills involve being able to (1) see commonalities and differences among different pieces of information, (2) link what is happening in one situation with what is or has happened in another situation, (3) distill large amounts of information, and (4) recognize what is key or most important. These skills are particularly valuable in the zeroing-in and working-out phases of the collaborative partnership, as described in Chapter 3.

Learning Styles

Each person has a particular learning style. By **learning style** we mean the ways in which an individual acquires and comes to an understanding of how something fits and operates in the world (McKeachie, 1999). For example, some people learn best by observing, some by reading about and researching a topic, and yet others by being told or by listening to an explanation. Some learn by doing for themselves, others by trial and error, and still others by being shown. What is important in a collaborative partnership is the "fit" between the learning styles of the partners. The nurse needs to be aware of her own learning and teaching style and the person's learning style, and then needs to modify her style to fit the person's. Nurse Cindy Dalton explains: *"The way that you're going to discuss something will be quite different with someone who learns in more concrete ways versus someone who is more abstract and likes to reflect."*

Readiness

In a collaborative partnership, **readiness** refers to a willingness to engage in health work or make a change or change course (Murphy, Taylor, & Townshend, 1997), as well as the intention to act (Dalton & Gottlieb, 2003). Readiness also includes a willingness to enter into a relationship with the other partner. The readiness of both the person and the nurse is important in the development of a collaborative partnership. The person may be more willing to engage in a collaborative partnership when she realizes that something in her current situation needs to change and when the benefits of change outweigh the benefits of maintaining the status quo. Three indicators can be used to assess readiness: (1) intending to take action, (2) having a plan of action, and (3) deciding the benefits of change outweigh cost. Intending to take action refers to the person's desire for change. Having a plan of action refers to having a concrete plan or direction in which to proceed when working towards change. The last indicator of readiness is based on the extent to which the person believes that the benefits of changing outweigh the benefits of not changing. When all three indicators are present, the person is in a high state of readiness.

Although many nurses think about readiness in terms of the person's readiness, this idea also applies to the nurse. The nurse may not be ready for a variety of reasons. Readiness can be affected by the nurse's level of comfort with what is of concern to the person. For example, the nurse may not be comfortable discussing death or issues related to sexuality and, therefore, may avoid these topics. The nurse may also not have the knowledge, skill, or experience to deal with a particular health concern. It is important for the nurse to be aware of his own readiness as well as the person's. When both the nurse and the person are ready, then they are more likely to be able to work collaboratively.

Sometimes people are ready to collaborate with the nurse around some issues but not others. Take the example of Mrs. Soloman, an elderly woman who recently lost her husband. She was not ready to deal with her grief, but she was willing to collaborate with the nurse about how to deal with her disrupted sleeping patterns. Several months later when the full impact of her husband's death was more acutely felt, she was ready to collaborate with the nurse in dealing with her grief.

Communication and Interpersonal Skills

Initiating, developing, and maintaining a collaborative partnership requires that the nurse possess a broad repertoire of well-developed communication and interpersonal skills. Although good communication skills are essential to all relationships, they are critical in a collaborative partnership. In a collaborative partnership, the person is actively participating in determining goals, setting the plan of action, and evaluating outcomes. Moreover, the effectiveness of a collaborative approach is dependent on the richness, thoroughness, and broad scope of the information provided by the person. The nurse must be skilled at inviting and encouraging people to share their perspectives on their situation, to tell their story, to identify and describe their concerns and their theories about why things might be happening, and to identify different ways of dealing with their concerns or issues.

Engagement, active listening, attunement, and negotiation skills are fundamental and basic interpersonal skills that must be part of every nurse's repertoire. **Engagement skills** refer to the ability of the partners to engage with each other so that they can establish a relationship. It is somewhat similar to striking a match. If the match doesn't catch, then there can be no fire. People are more likely to engage with the nurse and to work in partnership when they feel validated and understood. They will feel understood if the nurse has listened attentively to them and can see the situation from the person's perspective. Thus, active listening skills are essential interpersonal skills for a nurse. Active listening conveys to the person that her perspective is critical within this collaborative approach to care.

Attunement skills are another subset of interpersonal skills that play a critical role in the development of a collaborative nurse-person relationship. Attunement skills include the ability to read nonverbal and verbal cues accurately and the ability to discern when to slow down or move forward (i.e., pacing) depending on what the person can handle. If the nurse observes that the person is overwhelmed or tires easily, the nurse may decide to slow the pace of care by reorganizing, giving the person a rest between activities, or by rescheduling visits with longer intervals between appointments. On the other hand, if the nurse notices that the person is highly motivated and eager to move forward, the nurse then modifies nursing plans to match the person's pace.

The nurse must also possess negotiation skills and be comfortable with negotiating, because a collaborative partnership requires that both the nurse and person come to an agreement as to what they will work on together (i.e., goals), how they will work together (i.e., who will do what), and what they will look for to determine whether things are working (i.e., desired outcomes). (See the discussion in Chapter 3 on the zeroing-in phase for more about the skills involved in negotiation.) The person's negotiation skills also play a critical role in the degree to which a collaborative partnership is achieved.

As the other partner in the relationship, the person's ability to communicate effectively will also influence the collaborative partnership. People need to be able to articulate and communicate their concerns, and this communication can take many different forms. Although some may believe that verbal communication is a prerequisite for a collaborative partnership, this is not so. Infants, aphasic patients, people with dementia, or people who speak a different language need to find a way to communicate their needs and goals. Although there are certainly challenges to the collaborative partnership process when people have communication or cognitive deficits, a collaborative partnership in some form is possible; however, creativity is needed.

Nurse Joann Creager, who works with hospitalized geriatric patients, described the challenges of working with a man who suffered a stroke, which had left him aphasic and emotionally labile. His emotional lability gave rise to violent outbursts that necessitated a sitter. Nurse Creager explains: *"After he had been on our long-term care unit and we got to know him, the nurses discovered that his 'word salad' speech was always 'word salad,' but the intonation of his sentences reflected what he was trying to say. After a month on the unit, most of the staff could communicate with him to the point that they understood what he was saying. To a stranger's ear, this gentleman's sounds were just gibberish. However, the nurses were able to pick up the intonation patterns and determine what the patient was likely talking about. Then they could use yes/no questioning to find out what he wanted to say and needed. With the reestablishment of communication, we were able to collaborate with this man. Although many people would say that's an odd form of collaborative partnership, I think it was very much a form of collaborative partnership because once we were able to determine his needs with this yes/no questioning process we were able to reestablish this man's control over his situation. Subsequently his violent outbursts diminished to the point that he no longer required a sitter."*

Physical and Mental Status

Collaborative partnership requires a high level of involvement, energy, and investment on the part of both the nurse and the person. The nurse's and person's physical stamina, mental well-being, level of stress, concurrent stressors, level of fatigue, and amount of energy are among some of the physical and mental factors that will affect the degree to which the nurse and person are able to collaborate at any given moment. Moreover, the person's medical status is an important factor to consider. A study of hospitalized surgical patients' perceptions of factors that determined their participation in decisions regarding their care revealed that how well or physically fit patients felt affected their level of participation (Biley, 1992). When people are acutely ill, although they may be able to participate in some aspects of their care, their level of collaborative partnership may be significantly reduced compared to when they are feeling better. In a more recent study, cancer patients reported that their physical and mental health were important factors that interfered with their participation in making decisions about their care (Sainio, Eriksson, & Lauri, 2001).

Similarly when the nurse is concerned with personal problems or work-related difficulties or is fatigued, she may be less emotionally and physically available to the person. The nurse and person, however, can have a collaborative partnership even though some of their encounters may not be as collaborative as they could be. (See Chapter 6 on the indicators of collaborative partnership for a further discussion of this issue.) Box 4-1 summarizes the nurse-person factors.

Box 4-1	Nurse and Person Factors Influencing Collaborative Partnership

- Beliefs and expectations about the self, the other, and the relationship
- Knowledge of self and the health care situation or experience
- Critical thinking skills
- Learning styles
- Readiness
- Communication and interpersonal skills
- Physical and mental status

RELATIONSHIP FACTORS

The third major group of factors to influence the level of collaborative partnership that will develop between the nurse and person includes various aspects of the nurse-person relationship, such as the history of the relationship and the goodness of fit between the two partners.

History of the Relationship

The history of the nurse-person relationship is an important factor that will affect the nature of the nurse-person relationship. The history of the relationship includes how long the nurse and person have known one another, their familiarity and comfort with each other, the level of trust that each has in the other, the kinds of experiences they have shared together, and the circumstances under which they first met.

As in all relationships, a pattern of interacting or working together (i.e., dynamic) is established early in the relationship. Once this pattern is established and reinforced in subsequent encounters—the more it becomes the modus operandi—the more difficult it is to change. Change is difficult once a pattern has been established because each partner has a perception of how the other will behave and an expectation of what the other is capable of giving. If the relationship has been a traditional hierarchical one for whatever reason and the nurse decides to change her approach to a more collaborative partnership, she may find this difficult to accomplish. The difficulty arises because not only does the nurse need to change her behaviours, but so does the person. This requires renegotiation of the rules governing each of their respective roles. Even though collaboration may be more difficult than when these roles were established at the outset, it can nonetheless be done if the nurse is committed to a collaborative partnership approach and believes that it would be in the person's best interests.

In other cases, the nurse may have always subscribed to a more collaborative partnership approach, but the circumstances under which the relationship began (e.g., with a critically ill patient) warranted that the nurse assume more power and take more responsibility in making decisions. However, as the person's condition improves, power can shift back to the person. This may require that the nurse coach the person through this change in their roles and ways of working together.

Goodness of Fit

Goodness of fit refers to the compatibility of the capacities and characteristics of one partner and the demands and expectations of the other. This is an important idea for nursing practice because it explains many situations in which nursing is effective or not as effective. When nurses are ineffective in a situation, it is often due to an incompatibility between what the nurse is doing and what the person expects, needs, or wants at that time.

The goodness of fit between the nurse and the person will affect the development of the collaborative partnership. For example, if the nurse speaks in a way that the person has difficulty understanding or is uncomfortable with, then the chance of a collaborative partnership developing is compromised. Or if the person has a great need for sophisticated information and the nurse is unable to respond in a meaningful way, then the person may not see the nurse as a credible partner and collaborative partnership will be less likely to occur.

ENVIRONMENTAL, ORGANIZATIONAL, AND OTHER SITUATIONAL FACTORS

Factors in the social climate and physical space in which the nurse-person encounters take place will affect the collaborative partnership. By **social climate** we mean the organizational culture in which care is provided (Cahill, 1998). This includes the values, philosophy, policies, and staffing realities and workload of the health care setting.

The nature of the relationships among health professionals in the organization can set the overall tone for how professionals behave in that organization. If people observe interactions between nurses and physicians in a particular organization that suggest that the nurse is powerless and lacks authority, then it will be less likely that people will be willing to collaborate with nurses. It will also be more difficult for nurses to collaborate with people because the nurses may feel demeaned or powerless. The hierarchical nature of the organizational systems in which nurses practice may make it more likely that nurses will embrace a traditional hierarchical approach to care rather than a collaborative partnership approach (Bottorff et al., 2000). In contrast, if people observe interactions between nurses and physicians that are respectful and collaborative, then it is more likely that people will be willing to enter into a collaborative partnership with the nurse. The nurses in this setting will be more likely to collaborate with people because they feel valued and respected. In sum, if someone experiences a collaborative partnership relationship, they then know how it feels, they know how to behave, and they know what is involved. If nurses in an organization are rewarded for telling patients what to do, then it is unlikely that nurses will enter into collaborative partnership relationships with people.

The organizational and professional structures within which nurses practice can play an important role in the nurse's ability or willingness to work collaboratively with people (Kirk & Glendinning, 1998). Even in organizations that support patient participation and involvement, hospital and ward routines may interfere with and affect individualized collaborative partnership. Krouse and Roberts (1989) argued that the health professional's position of authority and power in the larger health care system, and even the language used by health professionals, maintains the power differential between the nurse and person. Biley's study (1992) identified organizational factors that affected the degree to which surgical patients were involved in decisions about their nursing care. The rules and regulations of the hospital unit, such as visiting hours and patients' access to kitchen facilities, constrained or facilitated patients' comfort in becoming involved in decision making about their care. Look around your clinical setting and consider how rules send powerful messages to people about what role they can play in their care.

Another factor shaping collaborative partnership is the nurse's workload. Even if the nurse wants to spend time with the person, the staffing and workload might be a barrier (McCann & Baker, 2001). Patients have reported that they are less likely and less able to collaborate when health care professionals have little time to spend with them (Nordgren & Fridlund, 2001; Patterson, 2001).

The actual physical organization of space in a setting and the designation of space for nursing activities can also play a role in shaping collaborative partnership. For example, consider whether the setting in which nurse-person encounters occur is one where private discussions can take place without interruption. If there is no designated space for nurses to talk with people, then forming a collaborative partnership will be more difficult. The allocation of space for nurse-person encounters also sends a powerful covert message about the importance and value of nursing care to the organization. Chan's study (2003) of nurse-teenager encounters in an ambulatory chronic illness care setting found that lack of private, designated space for nurses to explore teenagers' concerns resulted in many teens' concerns not being addressed.

Attributes of the physical environment may affect the development of collaborative partnership. Parents of critically ill children found it easier to communicate and connect with nurses in less acute care wards than they did when their child was in the highly technical setting (Espezel & Canam, 2003).

All of the nurse, person, and environmental factors are to varying degrees influenced by the larger social, cultural, political, and historical contexts in which the collaborative relationship is situated. In Chapter 1, we briefly discussed the forces that have given rise to a collaborative partnership approach within the current health care system. It is important to keep in mind that less obvious larger environmental factors shape the nature and form that the collaborative partnership takes. For example, during the Toronto and Hong Kong SARS outbreak of 2003, patients were placed in protective isolation, nurses wore protective garments, and family visiting was all but eliminated in an attempt to contain the spread of the disease. Moreover, nurses were fearful of patient contact and health professionals did not understand the epidemiology of the disease. This larger sociopolitical context affected the organization and operation of health care institutions, and this in turn obviously had important repercussions on how nurses related to patients and on how patients related to nurses (Naylor, 2003).

HOW TO USE THIS KNOWLEDGE TO PROMOTE COLLABORATIVE PARTNERSHIP

The Collaborative Partnership Factors Assessment Guide Checklist on pages 68-69 can be used in two ways: First, it can be used to identify the critical factors that the nurse should attend to in order to create or optimize the conditions needed to foster the development of a collaborative partnership. Second, once the relationship has been developed, the assessment guide can be used to continually monitor the nature of the collaborative partnership and determine if and when the conditions need to be modified or reinforced to further the relationship. It is important to keep in mind that the factors that shape the collaborative partnership are in a constant state of flux and will vary over time. Therefore, as the nurse works with a person, he should continually assess the factors that influence collaborative partnership and evaluate the effectiveness of the collaborative partnership.

If the initial assessment reveals that the person is unable to easily communicate her goals and needs to the nurse, then the nurse needs to determine how best to facilitate or optimize the person's ability to do so. (See Chapter 7 for the clinical experts' discussion of this.) If on the other hand, the assessment reveals that the setting in which encounters typically take place (e.g., a busy hospital unit) is not conducive to collaborative partnership, then the nurse needs to find other locations for encounters or devise ways of minimizing the problems in the setting that make collaborative partnership difficult. If the nurse observes that the person believes that health professionals know what is best for her and that her role is to do what professionals advise, then over time the nurse may try to help the person see that she can play a more active role in her care and that there are benefits to her doing so. (See Chapter 8 for the clinical experts' further discussion of this situation.)

It is also imperative to consider which factors can be altered or enhanced and which of the factors are less modifiable. By working on the modifiable factors, the nurse can maximize the conditions that will be most conducive to creating a

COLLABORATIVE PARTNERSHIP FACTORS ASSESSMENT GUIDE CHECKLIST

Factor	Observation

Nurse

❑ Beliefs and expectations
- About the nurse-person relationship
- About the nurse's role
- About the person's role

❑ Knowledge
- Of the medical condition
- Of responses to health and illness situations
- Of collaborative partnership

❑ Critical thinking skills
- Ability to link, see patterns, relating pieces of information
- Ability to summarize information

❑ Learning styles
- How they best learn/teach

❑ Readiness for learning or change
- Intent to take action
- Plan to do something
- Consideration of how benefits outweigh costs

❑ Communication and interpersonal skills
- Inviting to share perspective
- Attuned to the person's feelings
- Negotiation skills

❑ Physical and mental status
- Involvement
- Energy
- Physical stamina
- Mental well-being
- Level of stress

Person

❑ Beliefs and expectations
- About the nurse-person relationship
- About the nurse's role
- About the person's role

❑ Knowledge
- Of his own medical condition
- Past and current responses to health and illness situations
- Of collaborative partnership

COLLABORATIVE PARTNERSHIP FACTORS ASSESSMENT GUIDE CHECKLIST—CONT'D	
Factor	**Observation**
Person	
❑ Critical thinking skills	
❑ Learning styles • How they best learn	

❑ Readiness for learning or change
  • Intent to take action
  • Plan to do something
  • Consideration of how benefits outweigh costs	

❑ Communication and interpersonal skills
  • Able to share perspective
  • Attuned with own feelings
  • Negotiation skills	

❑ Physical and mental status
  • Involvement
  • Energy
  • Physical stamina
  • Mental well-being
  • Level of stress	

❑ Relationship
  • History
  • Goodness of fit	

❑ Environmental, organizational, and contextual
  • Values, philosophy, and policies of care setting and leadership
  • Relationships among health professionals
  • Physical environment	

collaborative partnership. It might be impossible to change the leadership of a health care organization that does not value collaboration with patients and their families. On the other hand, it is possible to improve one's skill in inviting people to share their perceptions and opinions. Communication skills such as respectful listening and open-ended questioning are skills that can be learned and are important prerequisites for collaborative partnership.

CONCLUSION

This chapter described myriad nurse, person, relationship, and environmental factors that influence the collaborative partnership. However, these are just a few factors among many potential ones. The point here is that personal, relationship, and environmental factors affect collaborative partnerships in very real ways. The interplay among all of these factors determines the degree to which the nurse will be able to implement a collaborative partnership approach with the person and the degree to which the person will partner with the nurse.

Both the nurse and the person bring to the collaborative partnership personal qualities and experiences that affect the extent to which they can work together collaboratively. These qualities will affect the nature of their relationship, and the importance of these qualities will vary depending on the larger environment and on the sociocultural situation. Beliefs and expectations, knowledge, critical thinking skills, learning styles, readiness, communication and interpersonal skills, and physical and mental status are the factors within both the nurse and the person that will influence to what extent they are able to work in a collaborative partnership. The history of their relationship and the goodness of fit between the nurse and the person will also affect aspects of their relationship. Aspects of the environment in which the nurse and person develop their partnership will also influence the extent to which the relationship is collaborative. These aspects include the values, philosophy, and policies of the health care organization and its leadership, the nature of the relationships among health care professionals, and the physical attributes and design of the health care setting.

KEY TERMS

attunement skills   **learning style**
Collaborative Partnership Factors Assessment Guide   **readiness**
engagement skills   **social climate**
goodness of fit

SUGGESTED READINGS

Ashworth, P., Longmate, M. A., & Morrison, P. (1992). Patient participation: Its meaning and significance in the context of caring. *Journal of Advanced Nursing, 17,* 1430-1439. Describes some general indicators of patient participation in their care.

Biley, F. (1992). Some determinants that affect patient participation in decision making about nursing care. *Journal of Advanced Nursing, 17,* 414-421. A grounded theory study that describes hospitalized surgical patients' perceptions of the determinants of their participation in the decision-making around their care.

Espezel, H. J. E., & Canam, C. J. (2003). Parent-nurse interactions: Care of hospitalized children. *Journal of Advanced Nursing, 44,* 34-41. This qualitative study of parents of hospitalized children highlights many of the factors that influence nurse-person interactions.

Chapter 5

NURSING STRATEGIES FOR A COLLABORATIVE PARTNERSHIP

I talk about my role and ask how they see their role. I use the words working together, and I may summarize "This is how I hear you would like to be involved, this is what I can contribute, and this is how we can work together."
—Nurse Jane Chambers-Evans

After reading this chapter you should be able to:
- Have a greater appreciation of the ingredients of a collaborative partnership
- Recognize that any given strategy may foster the development of several of the ingredients of a collaborative partnership
- Outline a range of strategies and techniques that can be used to foster each ingredient of the collaborative partnership in practice

Although many nurses would like to work collaboratively with people, most are not quite sure how to proceed. They may have a theoretical understanding of collaborative partnership but struggle with how to translate these ideas into practice. They may be unsure about what to say and how to behave to promote the person's fullest participation in this process. To work collaboratively, nurses require a broad repertoire of strategies. This chapter describes a variety of nursing strategies that can be used to develop and maintain a collaborative partnership.

Recall from Chapter 2 that the essential ingredients of a collaborative partnership are sharing power, being open and respectful, being nonjudgmental and accepting, living with ambiguity, and being self-aware and reflective. It is these ingredients that the nurse needs to develop, enhance, and maintain to attain collaborative partnership. These ingredients are highly interrelated, which means that if the nurse uses one nursing strategy to promote one ingredient, the nurse may intentionally or unintentionally be affecting the other ingredients as well.

The list of strategies described in this chapter is not exhaustive. As nurses adopt a collaborative approach and feel increasingly comfortable using it, they will undoubtedly discover many other strategies and gradually add these to broaden their repertoires.

STRATEGIES FOR SHARING POWER

The collaborative process begins as the nurse approaches the person in a manner that will set the stage for a collaborative partnership. The stage for a collaborative partnership is set when the nurse works toward balancing power with the person. The goal of these **power-sharing strategies** is to give a message to the person: "Your perspective of your own situation is paramount and you may want to play a major role in directing your own care." The way the nurse conveys this message is both explicit, through the statements that she makes, and implicit, through the language, actions, and behaviours that the nurse deliberately chooses.

Keep in mind that every nursing behaviour or statement in an encounter with a person conveys a message about how power is distributed in the relationship and reveals what the nurse believes and values about collaborative partnership. Small, seemingly insignificant behaviours send strong messages. Take the seemingly innocuous act of sitting behind a desk. When a nurse sits behind a desk, what does this action communicate about the nurse's power? When a nurse sits beside a person, do you think that this sends a different message? If the nurse just gives lip service to the notion of collaborative partnership, meaning her behaviour and actions are incongruent or inconsistent with a collaborative stance, then the relationship is less likely to be a collaborative one.

Shared decision making is a hallmark of collaborative partnerships. Therefore, many of the strategies that nurses can use to balance power in the relationship are related to the process of decision making. In a collaborative partnership, the nurse invites the person to participate in decisions about many aspects of their work together, such as when to meet, what will be discussed, what needs attention and what can wait, and how to tackle a problem. We next describe specific strategies that nurses have found helpful for sharing power.

Use Language That Conveys the Idea of Partnership

The language that health professionals use in interactions with people reflects the power distribution in the relationship (Haug, 1996). The choice of words that nurses use to approach people, to address themselves or others, to explain a procedure or diagnosis, or to discuss decisions about care reflects the nurse's ideas about power and control. For example, a common practice that maintains a power differential between the physician and the person is that of the physician calling the person by his first name, but referring to herself as "doctor." Some nurses have gone the opposite way. The person may be referred to by his full name, but the nurse refers to herself only by her first name, thus diminishing the power of the nurse's position. In a collaborative partnership, the nurse should address the person by his full name and refer to herself by her full name as well.

The way in which nurses use medical terminology and language may enhance the power differential between themselves and the person. Patterson's study (2001) of people living with diabetes found that when health professionals spoke in medical terms that the patient did not understand, the patients felt that this accentuated the professional's power and distanced the professional from them. In a collaborative partnership relationship, the nurse should assess the person's knowledge of medical terminology and use language that is appropriate to the person's level of education, experience, and knowledge.

One way in which the nurse can convey the message to people that power is shared in the relationship is to use the word *we* (referring to himself, the person, and the person's family) to refer to who will be involved in the process, who will be making the decisions, and who will be doing the work. Especially during the first few encounters between the nurse and person, the nurse can make statements such as "We will be working together around this particular concern that you're bringing up" or "We will try to find out how best to deal with this."

The use of analogies that resonate with the person can be a very effective way to convey this concept of collaboration. For example, the nurse might say "We are in this together," "I am here to help you find out how best to manage . . . ," or "I will be walking beside you during this experience." When the nurse finds herself in situations where she feels that the person is not actively participating and wants to make the person aware of this imbalance of power, she could use the analogy that she feels that she is "pulling the person along" rather than "walking together side by side." This latter strategy should only be used when the relationship with the person is well established and the person trusts and knows that the nurse respects him and is in his corner. When selecting an analogy or metaphor to use, the most effective ones will be ones that have some meaning, familiarity, or importance to the person. For example, when working with a businessperson, use business language and metaphors (i.e., joint partnership), whereas a farming family would best identify with metaphors from their world.

Explain the Collaborative Partnership Approach and Its Benefits

Nurses should talk explicitly with the persons they are nursing about their collaborative approach to care. Nurses should describe their role and the role of the person, explaining that the work will be joint and that the person has an important role to play in the work that is being undertaken. Cancer patients have reported that they did not always understand what the professionals expected of them, thus they thought that health professionals should explain to them that patients can have a say concerning their care (Sainio, Eriksson, & Lauri, 2001). This may be particularly important with those people who want to partner with health care professionals to determine their care, but who feel unable to express their opinions to health professionals or unsure of how they could do so (Roberts, 2002).

The nurse might say, "Many people have told me how much they like working with me to decide how to manage their illness. So my approach will be to have you play an active role in your care. What do you think about this?" The nurse should also explicitly discuss the roles and responsibilities of each partner. Recall that a good collaborative partnership is built on the notion that each partner has a clear understanding of his or her own role and responsibilities as well as those of his or her partner. A collaborative partnership works best when there is a clear delineation between what the nurse will do and what the person will do. In delineating roles and responsibilities it is important for the nurse to explain his own role and expertise and what the person can expect from him. It is also important to make explicit the nurse's expectations of the person's role and to find out what the person's expectations are of the nurse and the person's expectations regarding her own involvement. This explicit discussion can allow the nurse to effectively tailor the collaborative partnership to best suit the individual person. Open discussion and negotiation of the person's involvement in decision making about the nursing care is thought to result in greater satisfaction and comfort in the relationship for both the person and the nurse (Walker & Dewar, 2001). Nurse Jane Chambers-Evans, a clinical nurse specialist in critical care nursing, explained that in the intensive care unit, *"I talk about my role and ask people about how they see their role. I use the words working together or making decisions together. I may summarize this discussion by saying 'This is what I hear about how you would like to be involved, this is what I contribute, and this is how we can begin to work together.'"*

Actively Elicit the Person's Opinions or Perspective

When adopting a collaborative partnership approach, the nurse pays careful attention to the opinions and perspectives of the person (Lenrow & Burch, 1981). Because the nurse knows that how people view a situation will affect how they behave, the nurse should begin by asking, "Tell me how you see the situation." "Why do you think this is happening?" or "Help me to understand how you see this." The nurse can also ask, "What things do you think might work or might not work?" or "What things helped in what we did together?"

The nurse also needs to use strategies that can amplify, elaborate, and interpret the information that people use to construct their understanding of the situation. Try questions such as "Did I hear you mention briefly that your husband was also ill? Can you tell me more about that?" (elaboration) or "What other ways are there of looking at this situation?" (interpretation). All of these strategies not only have the effect of obtaining the person's perspective, but they also help people get in touch with their feelings and ideas. Getting in touch with feelings and ideas and putting these into words and voicing them are necessary conditions for having power in the collaborative partnership.

Actively Share Your Opinions or Perspective

In keeping with the preceding idea, in a collaborative partnership, the nurse helps the person understand that there might be other perspectives on the situation. The nurse might say, "Another way of seeing this situation is . . ." or "Another person might see the same situation in a different way. . . . Have you ever thought of it in that way?" The timing of when the nurse decides to share her perspective needs to be carefully considered within the overall context and history of the relationship (see later section on being open and respectful). A delicate balance exists between how much of one's opinions to share and when to share it. If the nurse is unclear about how and why she is sharing her perspective, she runs the risk of undoing what she is trying to accomplish. Sharing one's perspective too early may make the person feel diminished or overwhelmed, thus, defeating the intent of the nurse's actions.

Invite the Person to Share in the Control of the Flow of Information

Sharing power requires **sharing information.** The person that has or controls the information is in a more powerful position than the person who does not. When the nurse operates within a traditional hierarchical model, the nurse collects the information and controls its flow. This is done by spending a significant amount of time asking questions and by being the one who asks most of the questions. An observational study of the interactions of home visiting nurses and their clients revealed that there were long sequences in home visits in which nurses acted as questioners and the clients acted as answerers; this pattern gave control of the interaction to the nurse (Mitcheson & Cowley, 2003). Nurses in this study and others (Henderson, 2003) also gave much unsolicited advice or information to clients in the form of suggestions or teaching, and would do so even when the client indicated that they had no need for the information. Furthermore, clients were only invited to ask their questions once the nurse had finished with all of his questions. Although this approach to assessment was intended to foster people's participation in the identification of their own health needs, it had the opposite effect.

In a collaborative partnership, the nurse utilizes strategies that enable the person to control the process. The nurse also understands that the person needs to have greater control over the flow of information. The nurse still collects information, but the proportion of time spent asking questions is significantly lower in collaborative encounters. The nurse asks open-ended questions to help the person tell his story in the way in which he wants to. In a collaborative partnership, the person should be involved in determining what information to share, when to share the information, how much information to share, and where to share the information. The nurse then needs to be sensitive to the person's nonverbal cues to assess the person's level of comfort in disclosing information. In a collaborative partnership the nurse might ask, "What do you think is important for me to know about this situation?"

Invite the Person to Share in the Control of the Pace and Timing of the Work

One simple way of sharing power is to foster the person's involvement in determining the scheduling of encounters or contacts whenever possible and when appropriate. In a traditional hierarchical approach, it is often the person who has to fit into the health care professional's schedule. In a collaborative approach, the nurse values and respects the person's time and schedule, as well as her own. The nurse also values the person's ability to determine the frequency and timing of their encounters. For example, the nurse might say, "When do you think you might be ready to meet again to further discuss what we have been talking about today?" or "Are you feeling that you are ready at this time to work on this issue or goal?" The nurse needs to exercise professional judgment to determine when it would be more appropriate for the nurse to make these decisions. People often exercise control over the pace and timing of the work in noncollaborative relationships as well, but in less obvious ways by choosing not to come for appointments or not following through on the nursing or medical plan. In contrast to this example, when nurses share the power of deciding on the pace, timing, and scheduling of the encounters, then the people involved have more of a vested interest and feel more like a partner in their care.

Raleen Murphy, a former graduate student, describes how pacing played out in her practice: *"A client arrived at the clinic to have his blood pressure checked. It was found to be above the normal limits. I offered a suggestion to the client: 'How about if we arrange to have you see the doctor?' The client firmly refused. To respect the client's wishes and contribute to peace of mind, I responded, 'Well, if I can't convince you to stay and be seen by the doctor, can I at least suggest that you come back early next week to have your pressure taken again? If it is still high, would you then consider seeing the doctor about your particular situation?' The client eagerly agreed to this offer, saying 'Oh yeah. I will definitely be back next week to have it checked now that I know it is high.'"*

Nurse Diane Lowden, who works with people living with multiple sclerosis (MS), lets them determine when they need to see her next: *"There are times when people living with MS feel well. That's a time when they use me less, because they need a break from the illness. They need a break from talking about it; they need a break from thinking about it. They will sometimes come in and see*

*their neurologist just because they're being followed for certain medical param-
eters. I'll suggest 'Would you like to meet today?' or 'Is today a good time for us
to get together?' If they are looking at their watch and say, 'Oh, I've got a customer to see,' that's my cue that maybe there's not a need at that time. Being collaborative means being receptive to cues that maybe they want to have a little
bit of a distance from our relationship. You still need to be ready to move back in
if they're indicating a new need, either around a critical medical event or perhaps there is something in their social or family domain that they would really
like to address."*

Determine Together an Overall Framework for the Relationship

The nurse should engage the person in a discussion to determine how they will
work together. Nurse Lucia Fabijan explains that she frequently uses this strategy in her practice with psychiatric patients: *"How about if we work together
for a period of X weeks, and then at that point we can look at what we've accomplished, what's worked well, and what hasn't worked. We can decide then if we
should go on with our work or not. We will work together as long we see fit."*

Nurse Fabijan has learned that determining a clear time frame is important to
assess progress and also gives the person the power to evaluate their work
together and whether the relationship will continue.

Engage People in Solving Their Problems Rather than Solving Their Problems for Them

In a collaborative approach, the nurse's role is to facilitate the person's problem-
solving ability rather than to move in and do the problem solving for them. Nurse
Jane Chambers-Evans explains: *"One of the things that I have to watch very
carefully is not to take on the role of rescuer, and not to take over to the point that
I am 'the be-all and the end-all.' People need to take some responsibility; otherwise, they do not learn the skills that they are going to need. In fact, there is a tendency, particularly in a crisis situation, for the nurse to just run in and solve all
the problems. People are not going to gain anything from that approach."*

Clinicians have found a number of methods or techniques that can facilitate
the collaborative problem-solving process, as discussed next.

Help People Explore, Identify, Clarify, and Prioritize What They Want

Nurses should structure a discussion or a series of discussions that helps the person explore, identify, clarify, and prioritize what it is they want to do, what they
want to accomplish, or what they need. Questions that can be asked include
"What would you like for us to work on together?"; "Picture yourself a month
from now. What would you like to see?"; or "I was wondering what you think

would be the best use of our time?" This technique was first described in Chapter 3 during the discussion of the zeroing-in phase.

The nurse should help the person to brainstorm or examine the alternative choices or actions from which they could choose. You may recall that the idea of brainstorming is a technique that can be used in the working-out phase of the Spiralling Model of Collaborative Partnership (see Chapter 3). Both the nurse and the person should generate ideas about possible alternatives; for example, "Let's try to think up as many different ways of dealing with X *(name the situation)* as we can. We won't worry about whether these might work or not. We will think about that later. For now, we want to come up with as many ideas as possible. You start. What do you think you could do?" (Later the nurse adds her own ideas.) If the person has difficulty generating ideas, then the nurse might start, or each might take a turn coming up with an idea.

Avoid Telling the Person What to Do

In some situations the nurse may feel the need to tell the person what to do, but this should be avoided. If a person asks the nurse what to do, one way of dealing with this is to use the technique of throwing the question back to the person. The nurse could state, "Often it is only the person herself who knows what is best for her. What do you think might be the best choice for you?"

As a partner in the relationship, nurses should give suggestions. What is critical here is when the nurse actually makes the suggestion. The nurse should first elicit the person's opinion before voicing his own. Other considerations are when suggestions are made and how suggestions are offered. The nurse should use language to convey that they are only suggestions that the person may want to think about. The nurse may preface the suggestion by using such phrases as "I wonder if . . ." or "Would it work if we tried *X*?"

Box 5-1 summarizes some strategies for sharing power.

Box 5-1	Strategies for Sharing Power

- Use language that conveys the idea of partnership.
- Explain the collaborative partnership approach and the benefits of it.
- Actively elicit the person's opinions or perspective.
- Actively share your opinions or perspective.
- Invite the person to share in the control of the flow of information.
- Invite the person to share in the control of the pace and the timing of the work.
- Determine together an overall framework for the relationship.
- Engage people in solving their own problems.
- Avoid telling people what they should do.

STRATEGIES FOR CONVEYING OPENNESS AND RESPECT

Openness is a key feature of a collaborative partnership. Openness is achieved through conducting frank dialogues in which each partner feels comfortable expressing his or her opinions. The nurse and the person must be open to each other. Openness conveys mutual respect.

During the early encounters between the nurse and the person, the nurse encourages openness on the part of the client, but the nurse needs to be cautious in expressing her own opinions and perspectives. This is because the person may not feel comfortable expressing his own opinions and perspective if he is intimidated by the nurse having expressed her own views first. If the nurse is too open in sharing her own opinions early on, the nurse may risk making the person feel that his view or perspective is not as valid as hers.

Once the nurse knows the person on some level, understands the person's perspective, and knows that a sense of trust has developed, then the nurse can be more forthcoming with her own opinions. Collaborative partnership, in some situations, involves sharing a very different perspective with a client, challenging his view, or inviting him to see something different. Nurse Gillian Taylor explains: *"A collaborative partnership is not just being nice. It is a process that allows you the space to share a different perspective. Whenever you share a perspective that is different or ask a question that may cause stress and worry, it is important to preface that with a brief preamble so that the question or opinion is not misinterpreted or taken the wrong way. These approaches only serve to heighten collaborative partnership."*

Although the whole process of collaborative partnership conveys respect, the nurse can use specific strategies, as discussed next, to further demonstrate respect for the person and their feelings, perspectives, opinions, and abilities.

Conduct Meetings or Interviews in a Private Location

Some people need privacy to feel comfortable disclosing information to a nurse. Therefore, the nurse needs to be aware of the person's need for privacy and attend to how the physical environment may be affecting the person. Once this is understood, the nurse then needs to create conditions that are conducive to facilitating openness. Nurse Jane Chambers-Evans finds this to be an important strategy for her nursing in critical care: *"You need to be able to create some kind of private space for the family. You need to create a space for discussion that conveys to the family that they have your full attention and that what they were saying is not public."*

Set Aside Time to Be with the Person

It is important for the nurse to show interest in what the person has to say and allow her to say it without feeling rushed. One of the simplest strategies to show genuine interest and thus respect is for the nurse to listen carefully to the person's story and to give the person his full, uninterrupted attention (Bidmead, Davis, & Day, 2002; Robinson, 1996; Thorne & Robinson, 1988). This means the nurse does not answer the telephone or allow interruptions when he is with the person. Interest is also demonstrated by what the nurse asks about and how he asks the questions. When the nurse inquires about events that he knows are significant and meaningful to the person, then this conveys the message that the nurse is genuine in his interest. Finally, showing interest involves scheduling enough time between appointments or activities so that both the nurse and person do not feel pressured by the lack of time (Jansson, Petersson, & Uden, 2001). As one palliative care nurse stated, "Act like you don't have anything else to do" (Bottorff et al., 2000).

Acknowledge Verbally and Nonverbally What People Are Feeling and Validate Their Feelings

Acknowledging what the other person is feeling has the effect of telling the person that you have correctly heard and interpreted his emotional feelings or state. Acknowledging feelings without passing judgment conveys respect. Nurse Margaret Eades describes a frequently occurring situation in her first encounters with patients who have just learned of their diagnosis of cancer: *"Sometimes you're trying to engage a person, and he may be angry, or may not want to see you. I am respectful of his feelings, and will say, 'You have a right to feel angry. Maybe this is not the best time to introduce myself. But I'm going to make this short. This is who I am and this is how you can reach me, and I'll come back.' By giving the person the message that it is all right to be angry and by being respectful and acknowledging his feelings, this often opens the door. Invariably, when I come back, the situation is usually a lot better."*

This example illustrates the importance of respect, as well as the importance of timing and pacing nursing actions to the person's needs at that point in time. In this case the nurse has not only acknowledged the person's feelings but has also validated the person's emotional response. Acknowledging feelings is a strategy that is not just useful with adults; it is also critical when nursing children. Nurse Gillian Taylor provides the following example from her practice with preschoolers: *"Part of the culture of pediatric nursing is a respect for the child. The challenge occurs when the child does not wish in any way to actually collaborate with the objective of the clinic visit, which includes nasty things. It's interesting to see what collaborative work looks like with a mother and child when a child, particularly under four years of age, is putting her mitts and hat on and heading for the door from the moment that she arrives. If I'm going to have a collaborative approach with that preschooler, I am going to show respect and acknowledge verbally and in my gestures the child's distress, frustration, and annoyance about what's going on. I may say, 'Boy, she's letting us know that she thinks this flu shot is a lousy idea. Confident little mortal she is. Look at her walking down the hall away from us; at what point do you think she'll turn around?' I use humour in this way to let the family know that I think this child's behaviour is normal."*

In this example, the nurse has acknowledged the child's feelings and put into words these feelings for the mother, reframed the child's behaviour in a positive light (i.e., confident and clear in communicating her wants), and in this way normalized the child's behaviour. This conveys to the child and family that the child's desire not to collaborate is understandable under the circumstances. Nonetheless, the child did need to get her flu shot, but this was done in a way that acknowledged the child's distress.

Identify and Comment on the Person's Strengths

Another technique that nurses have found useful to convey respect is to identify and note the person's strengths. This strategy conveys the nurse's recognition and respect for the person's knowledge of himself and his illness (Leahey & Harper-Jaques, 1996; Tapp, 2000). It is not surprising that this strategy has been found to be particularly effective. Noting strengths and commenting on them may help to restore the person's self-worth, which can be undermined in periods of stress and heightened vulnerability. It is during these periods that people are most often in contact with nurses. It also may make it easier for the nurse to work with the person, particularly difficult individuals. When the nurse focuses on strengths she changes her own perceptions of the individual. Nurse Lucia Fabijan observes: *"I identify every strength that I can find, and I comment on it. That starts at the beginning of the relationship and continues throughout. I think that, to me, is key. Because it often helps to broaden the discussion to other areas."*

There are several ways to identify strengths. The most obvious is to do so in a direct fashion by asking the person "What do you think you do well?" or "What do people tell you that you are good at doing?" (Feeley & Gottlieb, 2000). Another way is for the nurse to observe the person's behaviour, identify strengths, and share those observations with the person. Once strengths have been identified, the nurse needs to be specific and descriptive when commenting on them; for example, "I have noticed that you are very supportive of your husband when you tell him how well he talks to the children and is able to calm them down."

Explain and Convey the Nurse's Availability

Offering to be available to help the person conveys the nurse's willingness to be open to the person's needs. This can be done in a variety of ways. The nurse can describe the specific types of concerns that the nurse is available to work with the person on. Nurse Lucia Fabijan explains: *"The other thing that's very important is to be open to hearing people's questions and concerns around other issues. You should offer to be available between scheduled appointments that you may have set. I let my patients know that they can call me anytime and that I will call them back. And then, of course, I need to follow through and do it. That's a simple thing, but I think it's extremely powerful and that it really builds the collaborative partnership."*

Nurse Diane Lowden explains: *"After having made an offer to be available to work on how their illness is affecting their family and having explained how I see my role and how we might work together over time, it is not unusual for them to call me back three months down the road and say, 'Remember, you said that we could meet about X. I think I'd like to do that now.' It's like planting the seed of an idea and then waiting to see whether they're going to pick up on the opportunities that you've presented to them."*

Periodically Inquire about the Person and How He Is Doing

When the nurse offers to be available to the person, this puts the onus on the person to contact the nurse. The nurse could offer to be available and follow through on this offer by initiating contact with the person. When the nurse periodically "checks in" with the person and purposefully follows up on a particular issue, the nurse creates a climate of openness. It can be especially useful to time these check-ins to coincide with critical points in the person's illness or event trajectory. For example, nurses often "check-in" with patients when they make the transition from hospital to home or on the anniversary date of a death of a family member. Nurse Lucia Fabijan explains: *"I was working with a young man for two and a half years. We had reached his main goal and decreased the frequency of our contacts. I do remember some of his secondary goals though. I call him every now and again to see where he's at, just to check in with him. One of his secondary goals was to become more independent. I call him on occasion and say to him, 'I remember that you told me a long time ago that you wanted to become more independent. Is this still something you'd like to do?'"*

Not only does this strategy communicate the nurse's openness to work with the person, but it also conveys the nurse's ongoing interest in the person.

Box 5-2 summarizes the strategies that are available for conveying openness and respect.

Box 5-2	Strategies for Conveying Openness and Respect

- Conduct interactions in a private location.
- Acknowledge what the person is feeling and validate those feelings.
- Identify and comment on the person's strengths.
- Explain and convey the nurse's availability to be of assistance.
- Periodically check in to inquire about how the person is doing.

STRATEGIES FOR BEING NONJUDGMENTAL AND ACCEPTING

Recall from Chapter 2 that being nonjudgmental is another essential ingredient of a collaborative approach. Nurses need to adopt a nonjudgmental approach at all times but particularly in those situations that evoke intense emotion, either on the part of the person or on the part of the nurse. Early in the development of a collaborative partnership, some people may disclose intimate or painful information about themselves to test whether the nurse will judge them. The person is assessing the extent to which he can trust the nurse with personal experiences and feelings. Nurse Deborah Moudarres states: *"I find in psychiatry that people often come with feelings of shame and guilt because they feel that they've done something wrong. It's very important right from the start, in terms of both engaging the person and developing a collaborative partnership, to have a nonjudgmental attitude. With some people, there is a guardedness. They wonder how much they can reveal to you. The clients need to make sure that they can trust you. So there may be a kind of testing to see how much they can disclose to you and what you're going to do with the information. People look to see if any kind of judgment on your part is being made; that is, how accepting you are going to be about what's happened in their lives and how they're handling it."*

Nurses have found a number of strategies helpful in creating a nonjudgmental environment and communicating the nurse's acceptance of the person. In the same way that the nurse's nonverbal and verbal behaviour is important in setting the stage for sharing power, so it is in creating a nonjudgmental environment. We now take a look at some of the strategies for creating a nonjudgmental environment.

Mask Surprise, Alarm, or Shock

People may share with the nurse intimate details of their lives. The nurse's own value system or culture may lead him to feel that the person's behaviour is inappropriate. An inexperienced nurse may react with shock or surprise. However, being nonjudgmental means that the nurse will monitor his own verbal and nonverbal responses so as not to convey any judgment to the person. This is necessary if the person is to feel comfortable continuing to share personal information with the nurse. Nurse Deborah Moudarres explains: *"You have to learn how to respond to these situations. There are times where you would like to be able to say 'Time out, freeze. Wow, I can't believe what you just told me!' But you can't respond that way and be an effective collaborator."*

In other situations the nurse may be surprised by an unexpected behaviour and will need to monitor her own response so as not to embarrass or cause feelings of shame. For example, Nurse Cindy Dalton recalled a couple with whom she had worked for more than a year. It had taken some time to gain the couple's trust. On a routine physical examination, the nurse was somewhat taken aback to discover when the man undressed that he was wearing women's red silk bikini underwear. She knew that any comments or expressions of surprise could embarrass this man and undermine what had taken many months to achieve in building a collaborative partnership.

Do Not Pretend Not to Hear What Was Said

When a person divulges information that the nurse finds uncomfortable or embarrassing, some nurses may choose to ignore or pretend that they did not hear what was said. Other nurses may change the subject. The nonjudgmental response would be to acknowledge what has been shared by saying "I'm glad that you have shared this with me," "This must have been very upsetting for you," "I've heard this before" (if this is the case), "Sometimes other people have told me . . . ," "I appreciate that you are coming forward with something that sounds like it must have been very difficult," or "Yes we can talk about it."

Do Not Criticize

A sense of self-esteem facilitates a person's belief that he can act as a partner and bring something to a collaborative partnership (Kasch, 1986). Criticism from the nurse can only serve to undermine how the person feels about himself. A person who lacks confidence is particularly sensitive to misinterpreting benign comments as forms of criticism.

Purposefully Explore Feelings or Responses That Could Be Viewed as Unacceptable

In situations where the nurse feels that the person may be feeling something that she is hesitant to reveal because she perceives these feelings to be unacceptable, then the nurse might take the initiative to put into words what the nurse thinks the person may be feeling. By so doing the nurse conveys that these feelings are very common and that she understands what the person is experiencing. Nurse Jackie Townshend describes the following example from her practice with children who have cystic fibrosis: *"I met with an adolescent I'm working with on the ward while he was in hospital. I'd gone there to explore with him the impact of the disease on him. He had become depressed, and I was trying to explore how his chronic illness might be contributing to his depressed mood. I asked about his thoughts, about how much place his illness takes in his life. He talked about his treatments and gave me all the 'right' answers. So I stopped and said to him 'Because I'm a nurse and I work with people a lot, I know that sometimes they try to give me the answers they think I want to hear. It's okay if you want to say something different. Other teenagers have told me that they hate the treatments or they are a pain in the whatever. That is okay.' When I do this it says I'm not going to be shocked; I'm not going to jump on you; it's all right. I think that sort of reflects my nonjudgmental position."*

Box 5-3 summarizes strategies for being nonjudgmental.

Box 5-3	Strategies for Being Nonjudgmental and Accepting

- Mask surprise, alarm, or shock.
- Do not pretend not to hear what was said.
- Do not criticize.
- Purposefully explore feelings or responses that could be viewed by some people to be unacceptable.

STRATEGIES FOR BEING FLEXIBLE OR BEING ABLE TO LIVE WITH AMBIGUITY

Unlike other forms of nurse-person relationships, in a collaborative partnership much of the work that takes place between the person and the nurse evolves in response to the person's changing needs and situation. Furthermore, the person's situation may be unstable and rapidly changing (such as when a person is in intensive care) or slowly unfolding (such as when a person is living with a chronic illness). The relationship has to have a built-in flexibility in order to be able to respond appropriately and effectively to changing conditions. The nurse requires skills and strategies to deal with an agenda that needs to be adjusted and readjusted as the person's situation unfolds or her condition or circumstances change.

Understand That Collaborative Partnerships Are Not Always Predictable

Nurses need to understand that clinical situations and the direction that the collaborative partnership work can take cannot be controlled and are not always predictable. First and foremost, the nurse has to come to the collaborative partnership knowing that the only thing that is predictable is that people and clinical situations are unpredictable. So many things intervene in people's lives that even though the person might intend on acting in one way, circumstances may cause him to react in another way.

Be Willing to Take Cues from the People You Are Nursing

Nurses should be willing to take cues from the people they are nursing and "shift gears" when the situation indicates that another course of action should be taken instead of the current one. The best way to work within a collaborative relationship is to be open to what people bring to the relationship and to be able to adapt and respond accordingly. Nurse Heather Hart explains it in this way: *"If you're really going to work collaboratively with patients or families, you have to take cues from them. They're going to determine the course of your work as much as you are, maybe more, probably more. So you can't go in with a fixed idea of what the outcome is going to be. The outcome isn't always clear as you work with patients. It changes too because life goes on or things happen. You just have to be willing to have that kind of flexibility, and be willing to risk that or be open to the fact that it's not all clear from the start."*

Box 5-4 lists strategies for living with ambiguity.

Box 5-4	Strategies for Living with Ambiguity

- Understand that collaborative partnership work cannot be controlled and is unpredictable.
- Be willing to take cues from others and change directions if indicated.

STRATEGIES FOR BEING SELF-AWARE AND REFLECTIVE

A successful partnership requires not only awareness of the other person, but also an awareness of self. Self-awareness involves an understanding of how the situation is affecting the nurse and how the nurse's behaviour is affecting the other person. Self-awareness requires an understanding of the dynamics of what is going on within the relationship and continuous monitoring of this. Self-awareness is acquired through the process of self-reflection. Another term used for self-reflection is mental work.

Atkins and Murphy (1993) identified three key phases of this process of reflection: (1) having some awareness of one's feelings and thoughts, (2) being able to examine the situation critically, and (3) developing a new understanding of the relationship. Reflection increases one's own awareness of what is happening and helps one understand how her behaviour is affecting the other partner (Atkins & Murphy, 1993). In a collaborative partnership, reflection is an activity that both the nurse and the person engage in, and it can occur not only during the partners' interactions, but also after and between encounters (Greenwood, 1998). There are many different ways of encouraging reflection in nursing practice.

Engage in Reflective Questioning

It is important for nurses to ask themselves questions that stimulate their own thinking about the collaborative partnership. This should become a routine aspect of each nurse's practice. Each nurse might eventually create his own list of a few key questions that he can ask himself routinely to help him examine what is happening between himself and the person in a collaborative partnership. A series of questions such as those in the box below may serve as a useful starting point to encourage self-reflection. These reflective questions can be modified to best fit one's practice as a way of increasing self-awareness. Not only can the nurse use these questions, but they can also be used by the person to promote reflection (Robinson, 1996).

QUESTIONS FOR REFLECTION

Reflection

❑ What was I trying to achieve?
❑ Why did I act as I did?
❑ What were the consequences of my actions? For the patient and family? For myself? For the people I work with?
❑ How did I feel about this experience when it was happening?
❑ How did the patient feel about it?
❑ How do I know how the patient felt about it?

Alternative Strategies

❑ Could I have dealt better with the situation?
❑ What other choices did I have?
❑ What would be the consequences of these other choices?

Learning

❑ How can I make sense of this experience in light of past experience and future practice?
❑ How do I now feel about this experience?
❑ Have I taken effective action to support myself and others as a result of this experience?
❑ How has this experience changed my ways of knowing in practice?

Adapted from Johns, C. (1994). Nuances of reflection. *Journal of Clinical Nursing, 3,* 71-75.

Engage in Journal Writing

A journal is a written record of experiences, ideas, feelings, or reflections that is used to increase one's self-awareness, deepen one's understanding, and develop new insights. Journaling or diary writing can take on many different formats, ranging from the unstructured to the very structured. In the unstructured approach, there are no specific instructions, rules, or format, whereas in the structured approach, instructions are more specific and what is recorded is more focused. In either case, what needs to be encouraged is the expression of one's thoughts and feelings during a specific encounter. Heath (1998) has described a split-page technique that can be used. A page is divided into two lengthwise sections. The right-hand side is used to describe the events and the left-hand side to describe thoughts, feelings, reflections, and analyses. This technique can also be used to analyze a nurse-person dialogue and give insights into the nature of the collaborative partnership.

Engage in Discussions with Colleagues

Another way of encouraging reflection and self-awareness is through discussions with others. A number of different formats such as small group discussion or one-on-one supervision or advising can be used to create a forum for the nurse to describe to others what is happening in a collaborative partnership. These forums provide an opportunity for the "storyteller" to reflect and for outsiders to share their perspective. The nurse in telling the story often has to do some analyses and integration and, during this process, may develop new insights. The other people who listen to the story are often impartial listeners who can make useful observations about the collaborative partnership. These forums should be scheduled on a regular basis and become an integral part of the nurse's practice and ongoing development.

Box 5-5 provides a summary of strategies for self-awareness and reflection.

Box 5-5	Strategies for Being Self-Aware and Reflective
• Engage in reflective questioning.	
• Engage in journal writing.	
• Engage in discussions with colleagues.	

CONCLUSION

A clear understanding of the ingredients of a collaborative partnership, the phases of the process, and the conditions that foster the development of the partnership are critical first steps towards nursing within a collaborative partnership approach. Although this knowledge is essential, it is not enough. The nurse needs a repertoire of strategies that can be used appropriately at the right time to move the idea from theory to actual practice.

Power sharing is a key ingredient of the collaborative partnership. It is not surprising that strategies to decrease the power differential between the nurse and person are most prevalent in this chapter. Without addressing the power-sharing ingredient, the collaborative partnership can never be achieved even when the other ingredients are addressed. How we speak to people, the language we use and how we explain collaborative partnership to the people we nurse, and the way we invite people to share their opinions and perspectives are important strategies for sharing power.

Openness and mutual respect are other ingredients of the collaborative partnership and can be achieved by creating an environment that preserves the person's privacy, validates the person's feelings and experience, recognizes and works with the person's strengths, and conveys an openness to be of assistance. Furthermore, being nonjudgmental and accepting is an important ingredient of collaborative partnership that sends the message that the person is accepted for who he is and is a worthwhile partner. Strategies for being nonjudgmental include hiding surprise, acknowledging what you have heard even when that is uncomfortable, refraining from criticizing, and purposefully exploring feelings and responses that could be viewed by some people as unacceptable.

Being flexible and able to tolerate ambiguity are also critical to collaborative partnership. This entails understanding that collaborative partnership work is unpredictable and being able to adapt to changing situations. Finally, a collaborative partnership requires some degree or a large dose of self-awareness that is usually achieved through self-reflection. Engaging in reflective questioning, journal keeping, and sharing observations with colleagues are useful strategies for increasing self-awareness.

KEY TERMS

power-sharing strategies   **sharing information**

SUGGESTED READINGS

Feeley, N., & Gottlieb, L. N. (2000). Nursing approaches for working with family strengths and resources. *Journal of Family Nursing, 6,* 9-23. An overview of the strength's approach; what strengths are and how to use a strength's approach in practice.

Heath, H. (1998). Keeping a reflective practice diary: A practical guide. *Nurse Education Today, 18,* 592-598.

Jansson, A., Petersson, K., & Uden, G. (2001). Nurses' first encounters with parents of newborn children—public health nurses' views of a good meeting. *Journal of Clinical Nursing, 10,* 140-151. Suggested strategies to use during a first encounter to create the climate for collaborative partnership.

Lenrow, P. B., & Burch, R. W. (1981). Mutual aid and professional services: Opposing or complementary? In B. Gottlieb (Ed.), *Social Networks and Social Supports* (pp. 233-257). Beverly Hills, CA: Sage.

Mitcheson, J., & Cowley, S. (2003). Empowerment or control? An analysis of the extent to which client participation is enabled during health visitor/client interactions using a structured health needs assessment tool. *International Journal of Nursing Studies, 40,* 413-426. Strategies that serve as barriers to collaborative partnership.

Patterson, B. (2001). Myths of empowerment in chronic illness. *Journal of Advanced Nursing, 34,* 574-581. Strategies that serve as barriers to collaborative partnership from the perspective of chronically ill people.

Chapter 6

INDICATORS OF COLLABORATIVE PARTNERSHIP

The litmus test of a collaborative partnership is whether the person believes and feels that he is a partner in the relationship and behaves accordingly. The same test applies to the nurse.

—Laurie N. Gottlieb and Nancy Feeley

After reading this chapter you should be able to:
- Appreciate the importance of assessing collaborative partnership across time and situation
- Understand that some of the same strategies that foster collaborative partnership may also be indicators of collaborative partnership
- Identify the indicators of collaborative partnership
- Cite three reflective questions that can be used to assess the degree of power sharing in the collaborative partnership
- Use the Indicators of Collaborative Partnership Checklist to assess the degree to which the collaborative partnership exists in the nurse-person relationship

Although health professionals may believe they are working collaboratively, this may or may not be so. Professionals may espouse notions of collaboration, but their behaviour may not necessarily be congruent with this approach (Greenwood, 1998). Walker and Dewar (2001) found that the caregivers of elderly patients were not satisfied with the level of their involvement in decision making about their family members' care. The health care professionals, on the other hand, believed in collaborative care but acted in a way that was more consistent with a traditional hierarchical approach. This chapter looks at the need for nurses to conduct periodic assessments of the collaborative relationship by examining the indicators that collaboration is actually occurring.

ASSESSMENT

Because it is possible to favour a collaborative approach without actually achieving collaboration, at different points in the relationship with a person, the nurse should systematically reflect on the nature of their relationship. This **assessment** of the collaborative partnership is an ongoing process that occurs over the course of the relationship: before an encounter, during an encounter, and after an encounter. An assessment of the collaborative partnership is important because it allows the nurse to make minor or major adjustments in the way the nurse interacts with the person. The idea of assessing a situation is constantly in play. Just as individuals continually assess the temperature to determine what clothing they should wear, similarly, the collaborative partnership needs to be monitored to determine whether adjustments need to be made and what adjustments are required.

Various signs can be examined to determine whether a nurse and person are working together collaboratively. These signs are the **indicators** of a collaborative partnership. Therefore, an assessment should look for the indicators of whether (1) the nurse's approach is collaborative and (2) the person is collaborating. Both the nurse and the person should be involved in this assessment. The nurse should reflect on the relationship, and the person should also be asked to describe his experience with collaboration.

Many things take place in any nurse-person encounter. The nurse must consider and attend to the person's physical health status, the medical condition and its treatment, and the person's response to the medical condition and that of their family members, just to mention but a few. In addition to all of these many and complex considerations, when operationalizing a collaborative partnership approach, the nurse must keep at the forefront how the collaborative partnership is taking shape and developing.

Before a first encounter, the nurse needs to consider how to develop a collaborative partnership with the person. The nurse might ask herself: What do I need to know about this person to determine to what extent he wants to be involved in his care? If the relationship is already established, then the nurse needs to consider how to support the person's desired level of involvement in his care. A question that the nurse might ask is this: What should I say or do to promote the person's desired level of involvement in this encounter?

During an encounter, the nurse has to periodically assess the nature of the partnership. Questions that the nurse might ask herself during encounters include these: How are things going? What is happening?

After an encounter, the nurse needs to reflect back over what transpired to determine how well the encounter went with respect to collaboration. The nurse might ask herself: Do I know how much the person wanted to be involved or to participate? Did I give the person enough encouragement to participate in the way he wanted to be involved? In which ways did I support or encourage involvement in the decisions? Could I have done anything more? What other approaches could I have used?

Before we discuss the different indicators of a collaborative partnership, a few points need to be underscored. First, one indicator alone should not be taken as evidence of a collaborative partnership. Any single behaviour or indicator needs to be examined in the context of the whole relationship.

Second, a nurse's behaviour is a reflection of his beliefs and approach to practice. Many of the strategies described in Chapter 5, which the nurse uses to work in a collaborative way, can also be taken as indicators of collaborative partnership. For example, when the nurse does not change the topic after a person divulges sensitive or painful information, the nurse is behaving in a nonjudgmental way. This strategy to create a nonjudgmental environment can also be taken as an indicator of a collaborative approach.

Third, the assessment should consider the degree to which collaborative partnership is taking place in specific encounters and the degree to which the relationship is collaborative. In some encounters the relationship may be less collaborative, yet an assessment of the relationship over time could lead to a very different conclusion. Ultimately, the "litmus test" of whether there is a collaborative partnership is the degree to which the person (1) believes and feels that she is a partner in the relationship and (2) behaves accordingly by being actively involved in decision making at a level with which she feels comfortable.

INDICATORS

In the early stages of a relationship, some of the indicators of collaborative partnership may actually be just indicators that the person has engaged with the nurse rather than that they are working collaboratively. To systematically assess what is going on in their relationship, the nurse needs to know the indicators of collaborative partnership. The following list of key indicators is not exhaustive.

Indicators of Power Sharing

The key ingredients of a collaborative approach were discussed in Chapter 2 and the most important ingredient was how power is shared. Later in Chapter 5, we described the many strategies that nurses use to share power. It then follows that one of the key indicators of a collaborative partnership is the degree to which the nurse shares power and the degree to which the person assumes power. What are some of the indicators that power is being shared? What are some of the indicators that power is being assumed?

Power sharing is reflected at every phase and in every aspect of the collaborative process. The degree to which power is shared will be evidenced in decision making, from deciding on what goals are to be worked on, to when this will occur, and how it will occur. Power sharing will also be evident in how information is exchanged between the nurse and the person; both partners will be contributing to the exchange of information.

Both Partners Are Involved in Decision Making

Both the person and the nurse decide what they will work on, that is, the goals to be accomplished or the "agenda," and how they will go about working towards the goals. In Chapter 5, we explained that nurses share power with people by encouraging and facilitating their active participation in goal setting or problem solving. Thus, one indicator of power sharing is that both the nurse and the person are involved in making decisions. Both will bring forth their ideas about what they think needs to be worked on and how to proceed. Nurse Cindy Dalton explains: *"You can tell that people are collaborating when they bring up concerns, ideas about how to approach those concerns, or generate possibilities in terms of how to change."*

It is easy to assume that if a person follows the nursing plan, then the nurse has succeeded in establishing a collaborative relationship with that person. Not so. Some people may comply with a plan that is determined exclusively by the nurse but this compliance may be short-lived. Research has shown that people are more likely to commit to a plan of action if they have played a role in designing the plan or treatment regimen or in customizing the plan to meet their needs that fit their particular situation. A study of the compliance of patients with hypertension to their treatment found that patients who acted continuously in accordance with their regimen of care had internalized the treatment plan into their daily lives, felt fully responsible for their treatment, and had collaborated with health professionals on a regular basis (Lahdenpera & Kyngas, 2001).

To assess the degree of collaboration, the nurse can ask himself the following questions: To what extent are goals being jointly negotiated? To what extent are the alternatives for action being jointly decided? How much is the person involved in implementing the plan of action? More specifically, indicators that people are participating in decision making include: (1) They participate in discussions to explore, identify, clarify, and prioritize what it is *they want* to accomplish or need. (2) They participate in brainstorming to generate alternative choices or actions. (3) They participate in helping to develop the plan and test it. Nurse Cindy Dalton explains: *"You can tell that people are collaborating by how much ownership they take once the plan is in motion. When people come back and say, 'We tried this and we've found this, or this worked to a certain extent, or this didn't work as well'; that is, if they have actually gone and tried the plan of action and come back and reported on the effectiveness of that plan, then they are collaborating with you."*

Sometimes nurses may be inclined to prematurely end their work with a person when the person they are nursing is a high-functioning individual who likes to take charge of his care. With these individuals nurses may feel that they are "not doing enough" or have "nothing to do" and, hence, have no role to play. This may be a mistake. The person may still need the nurse to reinforce his efforts, point out his strengths, and provide support. Nurses may also experience the same feelings when a person moves from playing a more passive role to playing a more active one.

On the surface a person may appear to be collaborating, but in actual fact is not. The person may have participated in the process of developing the plan of action together with the nurse, but then does not follow through on what has been jointly decided. This may be an indicator that either the person is not collaborating or that there is something wrong with the plan. Nurse Lucia Fabijan who works with people with mental illness describes this type of situation: *"When you've worked with a person over time and the person is saying to you that he wants to be doing one thing and yet he is doing another thing, or if he has not tried out the plan, this may indicate to you that something else is going on that you need to address, so that you're not working at cross-purposes with him."*

Both Partners Decide on the Pace and Timing of the Work

Another indicator that a collaborative partnership is taking place is that both the person and the nurse decide on the pace or timing of the work and the scheduling of encounters. One strategy that nurses use to encourage power sharing is to encourage the person to play an active role in deciding the frequency and timing of their work together. Therefore, an indicator that the person is collaborating is that the person is participating in determining the timing or frequency of encounters with the nurse. In the more traditional hierarchical approach, the professional usually decides how often to see the person, and the rationale for this may or may not be explained to the person.

In a collaborative partnership, sometimes the nurse may determine that she should meet with the person. Based on the nurse's assessment, the nurse may propose to the person that they meet more frequently. On the other hand, the person too may share her view that contacts should be increased or decreased. For example, Nurse Diane Lowden had a long discussion with a woman with multiple sclerosis about a particular concern: *"At the end of this long, emotional discussion I asked this woman whether she wanted to meet again to continue our discussion, to which she replied, 'No, not for the moment. Maybe later. I think I know what I have to do, I have to go home and talk to my husband. I will call you later this month to tell you how things are going.'"*

This indicator may be less relevant within an inpatient setting where medical care and safety considerations naturally drive decisions about the frequency of contact. However, in ambulatory and community settings, the degree to which the person participates in these types of decisions is a more valid indicator of a collaborative partnership than in the acute care setting. Nurse Lia Sanzone states: *"In our community setting, the most basic indicator we have that a collaborative partnership is in place is when people come back to see us. It may also be that they increase their contacts and use us more. They just keep coming back."* However, if people merely keep their appointments, this alone should not be taken as an indicator of a successful collaborative partnership.

Given that an indicator of collaborative partnership is how the decision making about encounters takes place, an indicator that the nurse is sharing the control of the pace and timing of the work is when the nurse deliberately sets aside time to explicitly discuss these matters. During such discussions, the nurse might explain the various patterns that their work together might take.

During certain periods, the nurse and the person may meet more frequently, particularly during periods of crisis or when the person is ready to deal with a difficult concern. There may also be times when contacts are fewer, such as when the person needs a break or is not ready to address a concern. What is important in a collaborative partnership is that an open discussion between the nurse and the person take place concerning the timing and pacing of their work together. The timing and pacing of their work together should be reviewed and renegotiated at periodic intervals. These discussions, however, should not preoccupy or dominate the agenda. At all times, the person's goals and concerns should be front and centre.

Both Partners Share in the Control of the Flow of Information

Both partners are active participants in the process of exchanging information. This means that both feel free to ask questions and to answer the others questions. The nurse asks questions to gain a deeper understanding of the person and his situation. In the same vein, the person should feel free to ask questions, raise issues, and give freely of his opinion. If a person gives minimal responses to the nurse's exploratory questions, this may indicate that the person is not collaborating or is not engaged in a relationship with the nurse (Karhila, Kettunen, Poskiparta, & Liimatainen, 2003). Thus, an indicator of collaboration is when the person readily participates in the exchange of information.

Another indicator of the degree of power sharing is that the person feels comfortable setting limits concerning the amount and type of information she wants to divulge. In a collaborative partnership, people should feel that they have some control over what information they share, how much information they share, and when they share that information. They must be able to say to the nurse, "I would rather not talk about that" or "I am not ready to think about that" or "We aren't ready to deal with that." What is important here is not whether people actually share the information but rather the degree to which people are able to voice how comfortable they feel about sharing information. In a traditional hierarchical relationship, people may indeed share information but may not feel as if they had a right *not* to share it.

Several signs act as indicators that a nurse is sharing the control of the flow of information. Nurses who share power tell people that they have the right to decide what information they will share and when they will share it. Another indicator that the nurse shares the control of the flow of information is that she encourages the person to control the amount of information divulged by verbally acknowledging this type of behaviour and commending the person for having done so. For example, when the person says, "I would rather not talk about that," an indicator that the nurse is sharing power would be for the nurse to say "If you are not ready to talk about it, you should not feel pressured to do so. If you ever want to, I will be here, ready to talk to you about that."

Both Partners Share Responsibility for Achieving Goals

In a traditional hierarchical relationship the professional typically sets the agenda and, therefore, feels responsible for the outcome or what happens. In fact, professionals often measure their own success in terms of how well people have complied with their plans and how effective their plans have been in reaching their goals for the people. In contrast, in a collaborative partnership both the person and the nurse share in the responsibility for what happens and for determining if they have effectively met their goals (Allen, 1977). The person, as one of the architects of the plan, also assumes responsibility for how things turn out. Nurse Irene Leboeuf explains that the nurse is probably working collaboratively if the nurse does not feel that she bears the full weight of the responsibility for whether the plan is working: *"If I am using a collaborative approach, I don't have all the responsibility for the outcome because we are sharing that. I have the role of creating a context for sharing information with my clients, but they are the ones who ultimately make the decisions about what will happen. I don't feel all the responsibility on my shoulders."* Thus, an important indicator of power sharing is that the nurse does not feel solely responsible for either positive or negative changes.

Box 6-1 summarizes the indicators that power is being shared.

Indicators of Openness, Respect, and a Nonjudgmental Environment

In Chapter 2, openness was listed as one of the key ingredients of a collaborative partnership. Therefore, another indicator that the person and the nurse are collaborating is when there is evidence of openness in their work together. Openness on the part of the person and on the part of the nurse is not necessarily

---

Box 6-1   Indicators of Power Sharing

Both partners are involved in decision making:
- They participate in discussions.
- They participate in brainstorming.
- They help develop and test plan.

Both partners decide on the pace or timing of the work:
- The nurse sets aside time to explain this process.

Both partners share in the control of the flow of information:
- The person participates readily in the exchange of information.
- The person feels comfortable setting limits about the information to be divulged.
- The nurse tells people they have control.
- The nurse verbally acknowledges sharing behaviour.

Both partners share responsibility for achieving goals:
- The nurse does not feel solely responsible.

---

exclusive to collaborative partnerships; instead, it may be evident in other types of relationships. However, one cannot have a collaborative partnership without some degree of openness. What are the indicators of openness on the part of the person? What are the indicators of openness on the part of the nurse?

The Person Moves from Discussing "Safe" Topics to More Sensitive Ones

The sharing of information of a sensitive nature within a collaborative partnership may be taken as one indicator that the person is open. Expert nurses recognize that when people begin to share with them information that is more sensitive or more central to their true concerns, then the person is investing in the partnership. Nurse Heather Hart works in a palliative care setting and notes: *"It's kind of safe for people to talk about very basic kinds of care concerns. In my setting, we can talk about turning and positioning or we can talk about what life is going to look like when the person is no longer a part of it. So I think an indicator of collaboration is the person's willingness to engage in some of the tough work, and the less safe or not-as-comfortable discussions."*

Nurse Gillian Taylor describes one example of a person sharing innermost feelings from her practice: *"One sign for me of collaborative partnership is when people reveal to me their struggles with something. I had a father whose son suffers from crippling arthritis. This father had recently been to his nephew's baseball game and found himself feeling 'ripped off.' He told me 'I don't know if my own son will ever have a fully normal life' and then he said 'I hope I'm not becoming nasty.' He told me that his son's illness makes him think 'Why did it happen to me?' I told him that I did not think that he was bitter, but that how he was feeling was very understandable. I told him that it has to be difficult to look around a baseball field full of carefree young teens when you have a son who has really bad arthritis. That's human and that's okay. Revealing this to me showed that we had worked collaboratively, that he could reveal his innermost thoughts to me, knowing he would not be judged."*

Both Partners Feel Comfortable Disagreeing

One of the best indicators of openness within a collaborative partnership is when each partner feels comfortable enough with the other to express divergent opinions and be able to work through these differences. Both the person and the nurse are able to share their opinions, even if they hold different views, and take the time to renegotiate a more effective way of collaborating. This is a strong indicator that the person feels comfortable with her power in the relationship and feels safe.

People are open to sharing their thoughts with the nurse when they say things such as "I don't agree with that" or "I don't have the same way of thinking about this as you do" or "We tried what we discussed, but it's just not working." Nurse Lia Sanzone, who works in community health, observes that people are collaborating when they can tell the nurse that they disagree with the nurse's ideas for their care: *"One important indicator that people are collaborating is when they're able to say 'Okay, you've asked me to do this, but I'm not accustomed to doing this. But I'll tell you what I'm willing to do.' That is an important indicator because you know you have an honest partnership; you're really working together. Oftentimes, because we listen to their opinions and work from there, the collaborative partnership is fostered and develops further."*

If openness exists in a collaborative partnership, then the person and the nurse will feel comfortable not only sharing divergent opinions, but will also be able to manage these differences of opinion and find common ground on which to build a plan. Nurse Jackie Townshend notes: *"There are times where there is conflict between the nurse and the family over an issue, and you have to be able to talk that out, be genuine, and say 'We're not agreeing; there's something going on; let's talk about it and work through this.' When a family can turn around and respond 'You haven't been responding to my needs' or 'I feel that you're judging me,' then it reflects their openness. It also indicates that they respect me and feel safe. If we can work through this difference, then the collaborative partnership really moves to a different level at that point. It's established then that we can have conflicts, but can talk them out and move onward from there."*

Box 6-2 summarizes the indicators of openness, respect, and a nonjudgmental environment.

Box 6-2	Indicators of Openness, Respect, and a Nonjudgmental Environment

- Both partners move from "safe" topics to more sensitive ones.
- Both partners feel comfortable disagreeing and can negotiate a more effective way of collaborating.

Indicators That Ambiguity Is Tolerated

One of the hallmarks of a collaborative partnership is that two or more people decide on the goals and shape the plan of action. This process takes time and the direction is often not immediately evident to either partner. Moreover, many situations are uncertain (i.e., waiting for a diagnosis) such that both the person and the nurse must wait for new information before deciding on a plan of action. Indicators that the person and the nurse are able to tolerate ambiguity and uncertainty are the following: Neither partner jumps to premature conclusions, and both the nurse and the person persist and maintain the relationship during this time of living with ambiguity. During the early stages of the collaborative partnership process, when the partners are getting to know one another and zeroing in on issues (see Chapter 3), the nurse and the person need to be patient and explore the person's concerns, goals, and readiness in depth in order to come to a clear understanding of how to proceed (Box 6-3).

Box 6-3	Indicators That Ambiguity Is Tolerated

- Neither partner jumps to premature conclusions.
- Both partners persist in maintaining the relationship during waiting periods.

Indicators of Self-Awareness and Reflection

Self-awareness and reflection are essential ingredients of the collaborative partnership because these skills are needed to continuously monitor and shape the partnership. A good partnership is like a dance. One partner has to be attuned to the subtle changes in the other. To detect subtle changes in the other, one has to have a sense of self-awareness or an understanding of how one's behaviour is affecting the other.

Both Partners Are Aware of Their Own Negative Feelings

The nurse and the person have an awareness of their own negative feelings and recognize that these feelings are an indication that something is amiss in the collaborative partnership. Intense feelings or uncomfortable feelings such as anger or frustration should not be ignored. An indicator of self-awareness on the nurse's part, in the context of the collaborative partnership, is that the nurse recognizes the importance of negative feelings. Nurse Lucia Fabijan explains: *"If I'm feeling frustrated, then I know that something has been missed in terms of my understanding of what the person wishes to accomplish, what his context is, or what he wants to talk about. If I'm feeling angry, then that's another indicator to me that I have to pay careful attention to what's going on in the relationship."*

Thus, when nurses experience feelings of frustration or anger it is time for them to step back from the relationship and reflect on what is going on. If the nurse becomes aware of uncomfortable feelings within herself, then it is likely that the collaborative partnership is not working well for the person either (Box 6-4).

Box 6-4	Indicators of Self-Awareness and Reflection

- Both partners are aware of their own negative feelings.
- The partners recognize the importance of negative feelings.

THE NEXT STEP

When arriving at conclusions about the degree of collaboration in any given relationship, the nurse needs to be cognizant that a single nurse-person encounter may or may not reflect the overall tenor of the collaborative partnership. It is the overall quality of the relationship, the nurse's commitment to and understanding of how the process of collaborative partnership really works, and his ability to operationalize this approach in practice that will affect to what extent the relationship is a collaborative partnership.

After assessing the collaborative partnership, the nurse may conclude that the relationship is not as collaborative as he would like it to be. In that case, the first step would be for the nurse to examine his beliefs and actions to determine to what extent the two are congruent or incongruent (Greenwood, 1998). The nurse may subscribe to a collaborative approach, but the nurse's behaviour may not be collaborative. Take the example of a nurse working on discharge planning with Mr. Davis, an elderly widower, and his adult children. Mr. Davis lived on his own until his recent hospitalization. The nurse asked the man and his adult children what they thought about his ability to return to his former living arrangements given his current state of health. The family told the nurse that their father was having difficulty managing his large home on his own and that this difficulty exacerbated his recent health crisis. Moreover, since his wife's death, the man had never had outside help and did not want anyone in his home. The nurse, in talking to the father, suggested that she would make arrangements for him to return home with a companion or help. The nurse believed that by asking questions and seeking the family's opinion on what to do, she was acting collaboratively. However, her behaviour revealed that she was operating within a traditional hierarchical framework and not a collaborative partnership framework, because she ignored the information that she received and developed a plan of action that was not congruent with the family's assessment of the situation. She believed that she knew "what was best for the patient." Her belief that she was acting collaboratively was not congruent with her later behaviour.

In addition, the nurse should examine what nurse, person, and nurse-person relationship and environmental factors may be influencing the collaborative partnership (see Chapter 4 for a full discussion of these) and work to maximize the conditions to promote the person's active involvement and investment in the collaborative partnership.

If on the other hand, the nurse determines that the relationship is collaborative, the knowledge that both the nurse and the person have gained from this assessment and review of their relationship can be used to (1) maintain and nurture their collaborative partnership and (2) further develop both partners' expertise in working collaboratively with other people. In the case of the nurse, her increasing expertise in collaboration will benefit her relationship with other people and other professionals. In the case of the person, this increased expertise should be reflected in the way the person works with other health professionals and in his desire to seek out other professionals who will work with him in this way.

Indicators of Collaborative Partnership Checklist

The collaborative partnership needs monitoring and assessing to determine whether adjustments need to be made and, if so, what adjustments. The checklist below summarizes the indicators that have been listed in this chapter, along with the strategies from Chapter 5 that are in and of themselves indicators of the collaborative partnership. This checklist can be used in practice to determine the extent to which collaborative partnership is present. Because the assessment of the indicators of collaborative partnership should consider whether the nurse's approach is collaborative, and whether the person is collaborating, ideally both the nurse and the person should be involved in this assessment.

INDICATORS OF COLLABORATIVE PARTNERSHIP CHECKLIST

Indicators of Power Sharing

❑ Both the nurse and the person use the word *we* when talking about either the relationship or your work with the person. Both the nurse and the person use and think about the notion of partnership.

❑ The nurse explains the collaborative partnership approach to the person.

❑ The nurse and the person explicitly discuss the roles and responsibilities of each partner.

❑ The nurse and the person determine together an overall framework for the relationship.

(Continued)

INDICATORS OF COLLABORATIVE PARTNERSHIP CHECKLIST

Indicators of Power Sharing

❏ The nurse actively elicits the person's opinions or perspective, and the person shares these.

❏ The nurse invites the person to share in the control of the flow of information. Both the person and the nurse share the control of the flow of information (i.e., amount and direction).

❏ The nurse invites the person to share in the control of the pace and the timing of the work. The nurse and the person explicitly discuss the pace and timing of their work.

❏ The nurse avoids giving advice unless asked.

❏ Both the person and the nurse decide what they will work on; that is, the goals to be accomplished or the "agenda," and how they will go about working towards the goals.

❏ Both the nurse and the person engage in working towards goals or solving problems (through discussions and brainstorming).

❏ Both the person and the nurse share responsibility for the outcome of the work and decide on whether the plan has worked.

Indicators of Openness, Respect, and a Nonjudgmental Environment

❏ The nurse shows interest in what the person has to say and allows him to say it without feeling rushed.

❏ The nurse acknowledges verbally and nonverbally what the person is feeling and validates the person's feelings.

❏ The nurse identifies and comments on the person's strengths.

❏ The nurse explains her availability to be of assistance with a wide range of concerns.

❏ The nurse periodically checks in to inquire about the person and how he is doing.

❏ The person moves from discussing "safe" topics with the nurse to sharing thoughts, feelings, or concerns of a more sensitive nature.

❏ Both the person and the nurse are able to share their opinions, even if their opinions differ.

❏ The nurse masks surprise, alarm, or shock.

❏ The nurse does not pretend not to hear what the person has said.

❏ The nurse does not criticize, but rather tries to understand the person's situation or behaviour.

❏ The nurse purposefully explores feelings or responses that could be viewed as unacceptable.

❏ The person and the nurse are able to deal with disagreement.

Indicators of Being Able to Tolerate Ambiguity and Uncertainty

❏ Both the person and the nurse do not jump to premature conclusions. Rather they continue to work towards understanding what the real issues are.

❏ Both the nurse and the person persist and maintain the relationship through this period of "living in murky waters."

❏ Both the nurse and the person understand that clinical situations and collaborative partnerships are unpredictable.

❏ The nurse takes cues from the person she is nursing.

❏ The nurse is willing to "shift gears" and change the course of the work when the situation indicates.

Continued

INDICATORS OF COLLABORATIVE PARTNERSHIP CHECKLIST—CONT'D

Indicators of Self-Awareness and Reflection

☐ Both the nurse and the person have an awareness of their own feelings and recognize that these feelings will influence the collaborative partnership.

☐ The nurse asks herself questions that foster reflection.

☐ The nurse uses tools such as journal writing.

☐ The nurse discusses and reflects on her practice with colleagues.

CONCLUSION

In this chapter we have described some of the indicators or signs that a collaborative partnership is taking place. Being more cognizant or aware of the indicators of collaborative partnership increases one's skills in applying this approach in practice. Knowing that both the nurse and the person should be sharing in the overall decision-making process, deciding on the pace and timing of the work, controlling the flow of information, and sharing the responsibility for determining and achieving jointly agreed-on goals results in more effective power sharing, the major cornerstone of collaborative partnership.

A person moving from a "safe" topic to a more sensitive one and both partners feeling comfortable disagreeing with one another are behaviours that may indicate that an adequate degree of openness and respect has been achieved. The ability to tolerate ambiguity and uncertainty is indicated by not jumping to premature conclusions and being able to persist even in times of uncertainty and stress. Finally, self-awareness and reflection are present when both partners are in touch with their own negative or unpleasant feelings.

Often nurses do not give much thought to the dynamics of their relationship with the person. It is just taken for granted. However, given that the relationship is a key aspect of nursing care, it is important for the nurse to give thought to what is happening in the relationship between partners. This is not to say that the nurse needs to be consumed with the relationship, but the nurse needs to be aware of the relationship and how it is operating. This process of examining the nurse-person relationship involves an assessment of the indicators of collaborative partnership. If the assessment reveals that the collaborative partnership is thriving, the assessment reinforces for both the nurse and the person the value of maintaining certain ways of interacting. On the other hand, if the assessment reveals that the collaborative partnership is not going well, then the assessment provides ideas about what specific areas need to be targeted to foster a more collaborative approach. Even the smallest insights into the dynamics of the relationship can have profound effects on what is transpiring.

KEY TERMS

assessment   **indicators**

SUGGESTED READINGS

Allen, J. G., Coyne, L., Colson, D. B., Horitz, L., Gabbard, G. O., Frieswyk, S. H. et al. (1996). Pattern of therapist interventions associated with patient collaboration. *Psychotherapy, 33,* 254-261. This study investigated a variety of therapist behaviours (e.g., interpretation, confrontation, clarification, encouragement, advice, praise) to determine if specific therapist behaviours were associated with better or worse patient collaboration.

Kirschbaum, M. S., & Knafl, K. A. (1996). Major themes in parent-provider relationships: A comparison of life-threatening and chronic illness experiences. *Journal of Family Nursing, 2,* 195-216. This empirical study describes three patterns of a family's participation in decision making among families who have a child with a chronic or life-threatening illness. The third pattern identified is one of a collaborative decision-making style between parents and health care professionals.

Chapter 7

ASK THE EXPERTS I: GROUPS, SETTINGS, AND TIME FRAMES

Our best teachers are the patients and families who can describe how they live their lives. It is important to realize that working with people . . . we're learning every day. They're teaching us . . . and we are teaching them.

—Nurse Lia Sanzone

After reading this chapter you should be able to:
- Appreciate that personal characteristics, situational or setting characteristics, and time play a role in collaborative partnership and describe how these can be dealt with in nursing practice
- Understand that there is more than one way of dealing with a clinical challenge

---

In Part II of this book, Chapters 7 and 8, we have asked our expert clinicians to respond to some frequently asked questions about the challenges inherent in collaborative partnership. Based on our many years of experience helping undergraduate and graduate students and nursing staff to nurse collaboratively, we have observed that students and nurses often struggle with certain common challenges when attempting to translate a collaborative partnership approach into practice.

Although these learners believe in this approach and have adopted collaborative partnership as their framework for the nurse-person relationship, from time to time they encounter situations or people that make collaborative partnership more difficult to achieve. When analyzing the basis of these challenges, we noted that many are related to the personal characteristics of the person, the characteristics of the setting in which collaborative practice takes place, and the time available for the nurse to develop a relationship with the person. These common challenges helped us to formulate the questions that we examine in this chapter and the next. These questions also derive from our knowledge of the nursing and social sciences literature. We know that personal, situational, and setting characteristics are powerful determinants of how people behave, form relationships, and relate to one another. In this chapter we highlight some of the particular challenges of collaborating with different groups of people, in different settings, and across different time frames.

THE EXPERT CLINICIANS

At the outset of this book, you were introduced to our panel of expert clinicians. These clinicians were selected because of their experience and recognized expertise. All are advanced practice nurses who have a specialized focus of practice and a specific population that they nurse. They have expanded knowledge and skills, deal with complex clinical practice challenges that require sound clinical judgment, and function as independent decision makers (Styles, 1996). These expert clinicians work with people dealing with different diagnoses (e.g., cancer, mental illness, multiple sclerosis), with people of different ages (e.g., children, the elderly), and in a variety of settings (e.g., palliative care, intensive care, ambulatory care, community health promotion clinics, and home-based services).

We sought the advice of our panel of expert clinicians on how they deal with the challenges of collaborative partnership. We determined which expert clinicians might best be able to address a specific question based on their interests, clinical expertise, and area of practice. Each question was posed to two or more experts. Each expert was interviewed individually and asked to address the question from her own experience. The experts were then asked to reflect on how they operationalize the principles of collaborative partnership. Our clinical experts describe their ideas about how they would approach each challenge, but through experience and practice you may discover other ways.

In this chapter, nine questions are considered. First we present each question followed by the answers of two or three clinical experts. Then we provide our commentary on the responses in which we make more explicit the concepts of collaborative partnership that underpin the clinical experts' responses as well as the theoretical foundations embedded in their responses.

COLLABORATION WITH DIFFERENT GROUPS

Question 1: What are some of the challenges of collaborating with people from different cultural backgrounds?

Response of Nurse Joann Creager, who works with elderly patients:

When the nurse is not from the same cultural group or does not understand the person's culture, then collaboration can be very difficult. There is potential for tornados. The tornado is the culture of the nurse when it hits the culture of the family. These little whirlwinds can start small and gather momentum if you are unaware of how culture is affecting the patient's and family's behaviour. When this happens, you need to pause, step back, and think about what it is that the person is doing that is really bothering you. The problem often stems from the nurse's lack of understanding of who the person is and where that person is coming from.

Response of Nurse Heather Hart, who works in palliative care:

Nurses require basic knowledge of different cultures and their rituals, beliefs, and practices in order to understand people's behaviour and needs. A useful approach that nurses can use to acquire this type of knowledge is to say to people, "I'm not familiar with your culture; tell me more about what I need to know" or "I don't know much about what your values are or your goals at this time as they relate to your culture, so how can I help you? What would be most useful to you at this moment?"

The nurse also needs to understand what the purpose of the belief or practice is, how strong the belief is, and what the costs are to the person if they do not follow their beliefs. The challenge is for the nurse to determine how best to support the person. I think this requires a bit of creativity on the part of a nurse. Where I work, people are in their last days or weeks of life, and one thing that comes up repeatedly is food. Feeding a loved one is such an act of love and care for certain cultural groups. Because patients often aren't eating in the last days, families need to find ways of showing their love and compassion in alternative ways. So I ask myself, "How can I help these family members still extend their love and compassion to their mother in ways other than food?" Getting them to help with things like mouth care, massaging the person's body, or just sitting quietly with them are ways of helping them to still feel useful, to feel like they're doing something and showing their love to their loved one.

Response of Nurse Lia Sanzone, who works in the community:

Learning about different cultures can be an ongoing process for nurses in any setting but particularly for nurses practicing in communities where there is a large ethnic mix. I work in a community health centre in the inner city where a large number of refugees settle when they first arrive in this country. People who have recently arrived from other countries often don't speak our language, and they are getting accustomed to our ways of doing things.

Our best teachers are really the patients and families themselves because they are the ones who can best describe how they live their lives. It is important to realize that by working with people from different cultural groups, we're learning every day. They're teaching us about their culture, and we are teaching them about ours. Every time I meet a new family from a different cultural background, I learn . . . . An approach that the nurse might take is to carefully observe people's behaviour and practices and ask them to teach you about what they are doing and why they are doing it.

Once the nurse has an understanding of the person's beliefs, values, and prac-
tices, then the next step is to determine how to collaborate with the person on how
best to incorporate these into their care. If the nurse is to collaborate with persons of
diverse cultural groups, then respect is the key to success. One way that a nurse
might show respect for a person's beliefs is to be flexible and accommodate or tailor
care to the person's beliefs and values, as long as there are no safety or health
threats that might contradict doing so. For example, in some cultures following the
birth of a child, the mother has to remain at home for forty days afterwards. I worked
with a family who followed such a practice. The mother was concerned about the
infant's growth and wanted to check his weight. Many nurses might expect the family
to bring the baby to the clinic to get weighed. A more collaborative way was to take
the scale and visit this family in their home. In the community, we would never be
able to work with people if we did not adapt our ways of working to accommodate
their cultural beliefs and practices. Collaboration is essential to working effectively
with people from different cultural groups. Otherwise we just would not get to where
we want to go, much less get in the door of their home.

The nurses' responses highlight the importance of self-awareness on the part
of the nurse in collaborative partnership, and the ability of the nurse to reflect on
the nurse-person relationship and interactions. Working with people of different
cultures begins with the nurse having an appreciation of her own culture (Lynch,
1998). Being aware of one's own culture lays the foundation for learning about
other cultures. The next step is for the nurse to get in touch with her knowledge
of and attitudes about other cultures. Everyone has preconceived ideas and
beliefs about other cultures, shaped by their personal experiences and the media.

It is evident from these nurses' responses that respect is important to be able
to work with people from different cultural backgrounds. Self-awareness and
respect are two of the key ingredients of collaborative partnership. Cioffi (2003)
noted that effective cross-cultural communication includes respect for and
appreciation of cultural differences and the enjoyment of learning about another
culture, having knowledge about different cultures, and understanding that culture has a major influence on people's responses to situations.

Bushy (1999) has described a continuum of four levels of cultural-linguistic
competence in how people relate to different cultures. The first level is **ethnocentrism,** which refers to a lack of cultural sensitivity on the part of the professional.
The professional perceives her own cultural affiliation as the standard, and all
other cultures are judged in accordance with this standard. The second level on
this continuum of cultural competence is **cultural awareness.** At this level the
professional has an appreciation of and sensitivity to the beliefs, values, and
practices of the other person. The third level is **cultural knowledge.** At this level
of competence the professional has knowledge of other cultures and uses this in
providing care. The fourth and highest level of this continuum of competence is
enculturation. At this level the professional develops cultural sensitive care in
collaboration with the person, and the person is a partner in planning care. Nurses

need to be at least at the level of cultural awareness, and ideally should progress to develop cultural competency to the level of enculturation.

One way of developing cultural competency is to expose oneself to different cultures through interactions, readings, and involvement (Lynch, 1998; Pender, Murdaugh, & Parsons, 2002). Another way to develop cultural competence is to do as Nurse Lia Sanzone suggests in her response and ask people to teach you about their beliefs, values, and practices.

Question 2: Is it possible to collaborate with people through an interpreter?

Response of Nurse Margaret Eades, who works with patients with cancer:

People who have recently arrived from another country may require an interpreter to communicate with the nurse. The question in these situations is whether collaboration is even possible. The answer to this question is yes. However, these situations require the nurse to collaborate with both the person and the interpreter. Furthermore, the interpreter needs to understand the nature of the collaborative process and needs to convey this information to the person.

When using an interpreter, the nurse needs to be aware of the possibility that the message he thinks he is sending may not in fact be the message the person receives. When working with an interpreter, the nurse needs to be exquisitely attuned to nonverbal cues, verbal nuances, or tone in order to determine if the message that he is giving is being received in the way that he intends it. In some situations the nurse can successfully connect with the person in such a way that interpreters are no longer needed.

When the interpreter is a family member, there is a risk that the message may be different than if a nonfamily member had been used, because nonfamily members may be more neutral. The nurse needs to understand the family dynamics; however, these may not always be clear at the beginning of the relationship.

Response of Nurse Jackie Townshend, who works with children with cystic fibrosis:

I worked with a father who used an interpreter at the beginning stages of the diagnosis. The father did speak some English, so we could communicate, but we wanted to make sure that the information that he received was accurate. After one or two sessions, he didn't want the interpreter any longer, so we tried to explore that. He said, "They're not medical people, and I don't think they're translating right." Then we just went on struggling, but somehow we managed.

I did a whole genogram history with a Hispanic mother because we didn't have access to a translator. It was just phenomenal, because we got through all kinds of data. This is a family that came from a Third World country, and this mother had brought her child through Mexico to here, with cystic fibrosis [CF], and had done that in order to get treatment. She had lost three other children to CF in her own country.

When I was doing the genogram and we got to that information, I was overwhelmed. Can you imagine the emotional impact of talking about this [losing three children to CF] through an interpreter? Somehow, with touch and whatever, we communicated and she brought in pictures of those children and talked about them. It was so powerful. I thought, my God, an interpreter would have been an impediment. It would have been a very different experience. We don't realize how much we cue into the nonverbal communication. It really comes to the forefront when there is a language barrier.

People from different cultures may speak different languages and espouse different world views. Often nurses deal with these linguistic barriers through interpreters. It is important to realize that the interpreter has her own perspective of the situation and might filter the verbal communication she is interpreting through her own personal perspective. Based on the theory of **constructivism,** people build their own perceptions of how the world operates (Mahoney, 1991; Siegel, 1999). They select and choose from what they are hearing the information that fits their view of the situation. Thus when using an interpreter, the nurse must realize that the content of the communication between the nurse and a person may be distorted (Lynch, 1998). Furthermore, when working through an interpreter, the dynamics of the nurse-person relationship are changed because a third party is now involved in the interaction and relationship. The presence of a third party significantly alters the dynamics of the interaction and the relationship (Ransom, Fisher, Phillips, Kokes, & Weiss, 1990).

The responses of the nurses to this question underscore the value of the nurse tuning into the person's nonverbal communication as a valuable source of information when working with people who do not speak their language. Egan (2002) has argued that professionals need to develop a working knowledge of nonverbal behaviour and its possible meanings and learn through practice and experience to be sensitive to nonverbal cues and read their meaning in different situations. Nurses' reliance on nonverbal forms of communication in these situations has been reported by others. In studies of acute care nurses' experiences communicating with patients who spoke different languages, when interpreters were not available, nurses relied on sign and body language to communicate (Cioffi, 2003; Reimer Kirkham, 1998).

Question 3: Do men and women respond differently to a collaborative approach?

Response of Nurse Heather Hart, who works in palliative care:

I do not think much about gender as a factor that influences collaboration. In my experience, the person's personality is more salient, and the fit between their personality and my approach. I will vary my collaborative approach to fit the person's style. For example, I have worked with men and women who are businesspeople who like a very structured approach. I tailor my interviewing and problem-solving approach to fit with their personal styles and preferences. I always approach the first interview in the same way and then, as I learn more about the person and family, I tailor my collaborative approach to what I have discovered in the course of that first interview. I find that the variations in how I work collaboratively with a person or family revolve around personality differences rather than gender differences.

Response of Nurse Joann Creager, who works with elderly patients:

My gut feeling is that there is a difference between how men and women collaborate. In my experience, men tend to be more difficult to collaborate with because they have a goal they want to accomplish. They want to make a decision and move towards that goal. Once they identify their goal, they see it as their process, and they don't want me, the nurse, to be involved in their process. Women, on the other hand, like to be engaged in the process of discovering what they want and how to get there.

One of the core elements of identity is gender. Gender identity influences all aspects of behaviour. Women and men are wired differently biologically and are socialized differently, so there is little wonder that they perceive the world differently, react differently to situations, and form relationships differently. Gender differences are reflected in how men and women think, relate, connect, and communicate. Tannen (1990) described how men and women process information differently and communicate differently. When women discuss problems they want understanding, whereas men want solutions (Allen, 2000; Steen & Schwartz, 1995). Thus, it would not be surprising if men and women responded differently to a collaborative partnership approach.

A few researchers have begun to examine whether there are differences in men's and women's preferences for a collaborative partnership approach and how they actually do collaborate. Although some studies that have found that women regard participation in decision making about medical treatment and nursing care as more important than men (Sainio & Lauri, 2003), others have found no gender differences in men's and women's desire for participation (Thompson, Pitts, & Schwankovsky, 1993).

Another factor to consider is the gender of the dyad—that of the nurse and that of the person. Most research has considered gender as an individual variable rather than a dyadic variable. There is some evidence that patients perceive and expect different behaviours from female nurses than from male nurses, specifically in the area of caring behaviours (Ekstrom, 1999). In a meta-analysis of seven observational studies of physician-patient communication, Hall and Roter (2002) reported that patients tend to be more comfortable engaging with, revealing more to, and being more assertive with female physicians than with male physicians. Moreover, in general medical practices, patients were more promotive of a partnership relationship with female physicians than male physicians. Street (2002) has proposed an ecological framework for examining gender differences in provider-patient relationship and linking these differences to a host of factors, including interactants' goals, communication styles, expectations, and the ability to read partners' communication. In a comparative study of communication patterns in physician-patient dyads of different western European countries, female-female dyad differed from the other dyads inasmuch as female patients talk more with female physicians compared to other dyad combinations (van den Brink-Muinen, van Dulmen, Messerli-Rohrbach, & Bensing, 2002). Open communication is a key ingredient in collaborative partnership, and dyadic research is an area worthy of further investigation. It is important to recognize that gender is but one of the factors that can influence communication and problem-solving style (Street, 2002). Nurse Heather Hart has alluded to the idea that gender may be secondary to the nurse's and person's personalities in shaping the person preferences for collaborative partnership. In addition to gender, there are many different aspects of personality that may come into play in affecting the collaborative partnership, such as self-efficacy or confidence, deference to authority, and shyness. More research is clearly needed to untangle the role of the person's as well as the nurse's gender and personality variables in collaborative partnership.

Question 4: If you are nursing a family, how can you collaborate with more than one family member?

Response of Nurse Irene Leboeuf, who works with patients with brain tumours:

The process of collaboration is the same whether you are working with one person or more. Collaboration with a family can involve more negotiation, because there may be varying opinions among family members. It may take more time to negotiate with several family members about what they want to achieve and how to achieve it compared to negotiating with one individual.

Collaboration really means that I do not have the answers and that people and their families have the answers. By asking questions of the family, I help them find an answer as to what is preoccupying them, an answer that is even better than the answer that I could generate. The family knows themselves and one another better than I could ever know them and they come up with the best answers. Collaborative partnership also means understanding that there is no one best way of doing something. Collaborating with a family means that I need to be flexible to help the family determine the approach that best fits their situation.

Response of Nurse Lucia Fabijan, who works with people who are mentally ill:

Students often wonder, "How do you work collaboratively with a family when you've got a particular issue and there are four different views of how that issue should be handled?" The principles of collaboration are the same whether you are working with one person or a group of four; however, the complexity of the work is greater when working with a family.

You need to develop a relationship with each member and encourage all members to participate in the collaborative process. There is so much more data to gather and analyze, and that is what makes it complex. The trick is to find a common thread or a link between what all the family members want.

First, you need to obtain the perspective of each of the members. Ask each member what it is they want or how they see the situation. As you listen to the family members expressing their views, it is important to remain neutral and not buy into one or two family members' views of the situation. If you want to work collaboratively with a family, you need to be open to all family members' views.

If you are trying to work collaboratively with a family and one or two people are doing all the talking and some people are less vocal, then you need to actively bring the less vocal members into the process. In these situations you could say, "There are four of you here. In order for me to get a good picture of what is going on, I need to hear from each and every one of you. If I do not hear from everyone then I get a skewed view of things and we may not make the best decisions in terms of how to proceed." Throughout our work together, I use a lot of "we" language. For example, "We are going to look at this together and see how best we can tackle this situation."

If there is a common goal or view among the family members, then you can move on to help them generate ideas as to how to get to their common goal. Ask everyone what he or she thinks can be done. If the family asks at this early stage for your opinion as to what needs to be done, tell them you need more time to get to know them and their situation. After having done an assessment and gotten to know their situation, then you can tell the family what you think based on the information that they have given you.

If on the other hand, the family members' goals or perceptions appear to be different, listen carefully to all of their views. Then summarize the views of each member, and check with the family that your summary is accurate. If the family agrees with this summary, then ask them if they see a link between their different goals or views.

If they do not see a link, then you can share your ideas about links because the nurse has some expertise and can certainly use it to help families make links.

Every step of the way you have to ask all of them what they want to do and how they want to do it. With all of this information, you really need to listen and be analytic to work collaboratively with a family. You want to ask them questions that get them to do the thinking and problem solving as a group using their strengths and abilities.

I was working with a particular family where the mother had difficulties with depression for a number of years and was shoplifting. Each member of the family saw this situation very differently and each had his or her own explanation as to why she was doing this. One member thought that the mother had a problem with shoplifting and she had to do something to get this solved. Another family member thought the couple's relationship was in trouble and that that needed to be dealt with. Another thought that they were "all nuts" and they were going to do their own thing. My role at this time was to take each of the family member's perspectives and weave these threads together in a tapestry. I then presented my summary to them and asked them if this is what they were talking about: "Is this where you want to go as a family?" I had to conceptualize what was of concern to all of them in a way that was concrete and that allowed them to agree on common goals. The negotiation of goals is a lot harder to do when there are four people in front of you.

Response of Nurse Jackie Townshend, who works with children who have cystic fibrosis:

Collaboration with a family is challenging at times and can be a lot of work! One common situation that occurs frequently in my practice with families who have a child with cystic fibrosis is that a parent asks me to tell their child to do something that the child does not want to do. One family member wants me to "fix" the behaviour of another family member for them. For example, a father telephoned me the day before he was coming for a clinic visit with his fourteen-year-old daughter. He told me that his daughter had not been taking her medications. He said, 'She's coming to clinic tomorrow but she doesn't know I'm talking to you. I want you to lay down the law and tell her she has got to take her medications. Bye!'

Collaboration in this situation means not responding right away to the request of one family member to "lay down the law." I need to think about how I will deal with this in a way that allows me to collaborate with everyone, not just one family member. How can I respond to the father's valid concern about his daughter's health in a way that does not alienate the other person that I need to collaborate with, in this case the teenager with CF. You need to do a delicate dance. Collaboration with the father would involve acknowledging his concern and worry and exploring his expectations. Collaboration also requires honesty and sincerity on the part of the nurse. You have your opinion and you need to make that opinion transparent and clear to the others involved. In this case, I had to make sure that the father understood that, although he wanted me to "lay down the law," I did not think that would work. I needed to maintain my credibility and integrity with the adolescent daughter and to collaborate with her too. I explained this to the father. Together we looked at all the possible options as to how to proceed. One option we came up with was that the father could share with his daughter what he had told me about her not taking her medications. Another option would be for me to discuss this directly with his daughter. I had the father choose the route that he was most comfortable with. You have to be able to offer options that you are comfortable with too.

Having secrets between the nurse and one family member usually is not a good idea. I want everyone to know what the agenda is (i.e., discussing the medication issue). The bottom line is that the parents want the nurse to acknowledge their anxiety about their child not taking her medications.

Friedman and colleagues (2003) noted that nursing assessment, planning, and intervention are more extensive and complex when nurses work with the family as the unit of care. Our clinical experts agree that the collaborative partnership process and the principles that govern this process are the same with individuals and families, but what differs is the complexity involved when collaborating with more than one person. It is not surprising that when you add another person to an interaction, the layers or numbers of interaction permutations and combinations increase exponentially. When there are two people involved there is only one relationship; however, when there are four people involved then there are six relationships taking place.

Question 5: Can you collaborate with people who are not very articulate or have difficulty expressing their needs or goals?

Response of Nurse Lucia Fabijan, who works with people with mental illness:

People have varying abilities to express themselves. Sometimes you'll hear nurses say, "Oh you can't collaborate with that person, they're not very articulate. They aren't able to express their goals." I do not think that is true. Obviously the greater a person's ability to communicate and to express their goals and needs, the easier it is to collaborate with them in some way. However, it has been my experience that you can collaborate with people who are less articulate. But these people present unique challenges. People who have a mental illness sometimes have a lot of difficulty articulating their goals. You need to work harder and longer to explore and help them to express their thoughts. I may start by asking many general questions, such as "What do you want to talk about?" or "What is on your mind?" As they talk, I point out strengths that I am able to identify. If I hear about less healthy behaviour, I will ask them if this is a problem for them or if this is something they would like to change. Some people will be able to respond to this general probing and exploration and eventually state what they want to accomplish.

Other people will not be able to say much or their goal may lack specificity. For example, they may only be able to tell you that they want to be less angry but are unable to say what it is that makes them feel angry. What I need to do then is to help them clarify their goal. This can be done by reviewing with the person the experiences or events that are associated with the angry feelings. In this case, I would go over the event with them step by step, blow by blow. At the end of this very detailed exploration, many people will be able to identify what it was that made them angry. However, with others I may need to share with them my ideas about what I think made them angry, and then ask them if my ideas and my way of seeing the situation is correct or incorrect.

Some people may ask you a question, and their question really reflects their goal. The information that you are seeking is there, however, it is presented to you or emerges in a way that is less clear. You have to listen very carefully to what the person is saying. Often goals are evident but they are not labelled as such.

When people have difficulty articulating their goals and I have played a very active role in helping them through this process, I always say to them after we have concluded our exploration, "I have asked you a lot of questions. Do you have any for me?" This highlights the collaborative nature of the exploration that we are engaged in and gives them an opportunity to play a more active role.

Response of Nurse Joann Creager, who works with elderly patients:

The short answer is yes but it is not always apparent. The elderly population I work with has significant dementia and communication is a challenge. Sometimes nurses are able to connect with some patients but not with others. It is a matter of finding the key, the little window that will enable you to enter the patient's world and understand the patient's perspective.

Let me illustrate. I have a patient who has had a series of strokes resulting in significant vascular dementia. This has been accompanied by profound changes in her verbal communication ability and bouts of extreme agitation. Nurses were having difficulty communicating with her and finding ways to manage her agitation. I decided to spend time with her to further understand her as a person and to find a way to communicate with her. Initially I visited her when her friends were present and learned from them that she had been a very loving and giving person. I observed periodic bouts of frustration even with her friends when she referred to herself in the third person. She would say, "She's not doing very well," "She has problems," and "She doesn't know what to do." We were all confused about who the "she" referred to. Unbeknownst to us at that time, the third person was the patient herself. When she talked in the third person and expressed distress about "she," this was her way of talking about herself. The stroke had affected her language centre. Her friends did not understand whom she was talking about and frequently failed to address her anguish. Once I realized that the third person was indeed the patient, I was able to talk to her about these issues. This meant that I was able to affirm her loss and show her what she was still able to give. In doing this, I reaffirmed her personhood. Moreover, I began to communicate with her in her language by addressing her in the third person. I knew that I had hit the right note because of her responses. She became calmer and could converse about these issues. Once you have found the means to communicate, you are able to collaborate. Collaboration means finding out what is meaningful to the person and working together.

Collaboration can take many forms, and can even be simply giving someone a choice. We had one semicomatose patient who had been in the hospital for six months. No one knew what had precipitated the neurological damage, but it was clear he would not recover. He would flay his splinted arm, which some nurses interpreted as an aggressive gesture, while others interpreted the gesture as reaching out. The evening nurse recognized that he was trying to speak. She started singing to him in the hopes of calming him down. He tried to join her singing. She also offered him simple choices—Do you want the light on or off? Window or door, open or closed? He gradually became more aroused and began uttering words. His first word when he became more alert was that nurse's name.

The examples given by the nurses underscore the idea that communication is an integral part of a collaborative partnership. Nurses are able to work collaboratively with people who have limited verbal communication or language skills such as infants, people who are in comas, people with different forms of dementia, or people who speak a different language. However, the onus is on the nurse to find a way of connecting and communicating with the person.

Once some form of communication is established between the nurse and person, a collaborative partnership can develop. Nonetheless, a collaborative partnership with a person who has limited communication skills due to illness or disability will look quite different from a collaborative partnership with a person who is fully able to communicate his thoughts, opinions, and preferences. Simple forms of collaborative partnership, such as giving the person a number of choices from which to choose or seeking his preferences, are possible with many people who have very limited communication skills or who desire less involved participation in collaborative decision making.

Being respectful is one of the essential ingredients of a collaborative partnership, as we described in a previous chapter. The respect that the nurses have for the people they nurse is readily evident from their responses.

Question 6: How do you collaborate with people who are unable to communicate because they are acutely or terminally ill?

Response of Nurse Heather Hart, who works with dying hospitalized patients:

Some patients in palliative care lapse into coma in their final days and are unable to communicate. However, because I knew them before this happens, I draw on my prior relationship and assessment of the person to continue to work collaboratively with them. I know what they wanted and the type of care they desired so I continue to work towards their previously expressed needs or goals. This makes it easy to continue to collaborate.

I nursed a young woman who always wore nice pajamas in hospital and cared about how she looked. She never would wear a hospital gown. So when she was comatose, I put her satin pajama top on her rather than a hospital gown. I did this because I had prior knowledge of this woman, and sought to continue to honour and respect her preferences and wishes.

In other cases, a patient may come to palliative care in a nonresponsive state. Collaboration in these situations is a bigger challenge, but my intent is still to collaborate in some way with them, and not just give custodial care and meet their physical needs. I still talk to them as if they were going to answer me. I ask questions and inform them of what I am going to do. It is helpful to spend time with the patients observing their behaviour and how they communicate through their body language. You can pick up subtle cues as to what may be helpful to them.

If family and significant others are involved, you collaborate with them. They can help you learn about the patient and their goals for their care. I might say to them, "Your dad cannot speak for himself. Had you talked to him about what he wished at this time?" or "How can I best help him?"

Response of Nurse Irene Leboeuf, who works with patients with brain tumours:

Communication is really important to the collaborative process, so it is really important for me to try whatever I can do to find a way to communicate with the patient. I nurse patients with brain tumours. If the patient can understand but does not speak, then I want to continue to include her in any family meetings. I will often ask the family if they think it is okay if the patient attends the meetings. If the family prefers that the patient not be present, then I will tell the patient that I will be meeting with her family and come back and tell her what we discussed. If the family agrees that the patient should be present, then although the patient cannot speak she can hear what others are saying, and I can observe the patient's nonverbal behaviour to assess her responses to what is being said. I also try to show the family how to continue to collaborate with the patient by modeling how to behave with the patient (i.e., seeking the patient's opinion, talking to the patient) who perhaps cannot understand what is happening. Speech therapy consultations can also be helpful to learn how to communicate more effectively.

One of the most common misconceptions about collaborative partnership is that collaboration is only possible with persons who are intelligent, well educated, and able to articulate their needs and define their goals. This is not so. Collaboration involves the nurse recognizing, getting in tune with, and working with each person's unique capacities and competencies.

The nurses' responses also highlight that there are different ways of "getting to know" the person (see Chapter 3). Interpersonal and communication skills are key to knowing the person (Roberts, 2002). When circumstances prohibit the nurse getting to know the person directly, the nurse is still able to get to know the person by using other sources such as the family or significant others. When the nurse has cared for a person over time, the nurse has the advantage of using her prior knowledge of the person to care for the person in a way that respects what the person would have wanted for himself. In a collaborative partnership, the person is always at the centre of care. The challenge for the nurse is to maintain the person's status as a partner even when his ability to actively participate has been diminished.

COLLABORATION ACROSS SETTINGS AND ACROSS TIME

Question 7: How does the setting affect the collaborative partnership?

Response of Nurse Joann Creager, who works with elderly patients:

I work in an outpatient clinic, as well as inpatient, acute geriatric, and long-term care units. When your practice is in a hospital unit, people are on my turf. It gives me a degree of power that you try to downplay when you try to work collaboratively. However, I know that if pushed I could rely on that power to some degree. You don't have that if you're working with people who are outpatients. It is very different in ambulatory clinics or the community because then you are on their turf. It becomes even more critical for the nurse to listen and pay attention to how the clients want to go about doing things. If people don't like what you're doing, they're not going to come back again. If you really want to get some work done with them, you have to find a way to discover what it is they really want to achieve and convince them that you can do it together. I think that's the biggest difference. It's clear that they're running the show, and you're fitting in on the periphery instead of the other way around. Strategies for power sharing may be useful, and these can be modified for use in different settings. In those situations in which the nurse works with a person across the continuum of care and settings, and has a prior relationship with a person, then the setting may assume less significance.

Response of Nurse Jane Chambers-Evans, who works with adults in intensive care:

As a clinical nurse specialist in adult critical care, I often meet people for the first time in a real crisis situation. Within a collaborative approach one of my roles is to help the family describe to the team who they are, so we're building a picture of who that family is, what their values are, their beliefs, their understanding of what's happening, and what's happened in the past. I am building up a picture of the patient and family so that the treatment team can understand their context and begin to be sure that the treatment options offered are going to fit the family's values and beliefs. That's how I see it starting, anyway.

Nursing, as a discipline, has understood that the person and his environment are inextricably linked. One cannot separate person and environment. People's patterns of behaviour can only be understood in the context of places and times that constitute the whole environment (Kulbok, Gates, Vincenzi, & Schultz, 1999). People behave differently in different environments because there are different sets of expectations and norms that govern behaviour. People shape their environments, and the environment affects their behaviour. Just as environments can influence patient's health, illness, and healing, the environment can affect the nature of the collaborative partnership.

The environment in any given setting in which nurses practice includes both animate and inanimate elements. The animate elements include the relationship and interactions among the people in the environment, whereas the inanimate elements include the physical space and its design.

Nurse Joann Creager's observations suggest that the distribution of power is most affected by the setting in which nurse-person encounters take place. The organizational culture of the health care setting, the physical design of that setting, and how space is used in the setting indicate how power is distributed between professionals and patients. In hospitals, nurses are familiar with the setting, are in their own territory, and thus hold much of the power. Even the most assertive person when hospitalized often feels more vulnerable and powerless. This is because the setting and its organizational structure and rules are unfamiliar to the person, and the person is dependent on the nurse for her care and safety. In contrast, when the person and the nurse interact in the person's home, the roles may be very much reversed. The nurse may feel less in control because the reality is that they indeed have less control (Jansson, Petersson, & Uden, 2001). The nurse is a guest in the person's home and needs to behave accordingly. On the other hand, ambulatory care settings share features of both. Although the nurse is on familiar territory, the person is also less dependent on the nurse for care and ultimately decides whether or not to keep appointments with the nurse.

In a Swedish study of creating the conditions for a long-lasting collaborative relationship between nurses and parents of newborn children, nurses identified the importance of taking into account the place or setting in which the first encounter took place (Jansson et al., 2001). The nurses thought that the hospital setting was less optimal than the home setting for connecting with first-time parents because of lack of time, the stress-charged atmosphere, multiple interruptions, professional status of the nurse, and the focus on medical concerns. Other studies of caregivers or family members of hospitalized patients have supported the notion that the setting influences how nurses and professionals behave and interact. Allen (2000) found that caregivers were less comfortable caring for their family members in the hospital and had more difficulty negotiating a role for themselves with nurses in the hospital setting compared to when they were at home. In a study to determine the roles of parents and professionals in caring for children with complex health care needs, health professionals reported that parents exercised greater power in their home than in hospital; however, parents thought that it was difficult to have power even in relation to their child's care at home (Kirk, 2001).

Question 8: Can a collaborative approach to nursing be used where nursing encounters are brief, such as in the emergency department or in a student health centre?

Response of Nurse Irene Leboeuf, who works with patients with brain tumours:

Yes, it can because collaboration is a stance or a philosophy that frames the nurse's approach to care. All behaviours, even simple behaviours such as the way you greet people, convey to people that you view them as a partner. I think the words that you choose and the way you behave are simple things that can be used to convey that you would like to work in partnership. I think I can convey a collaborative approach in a two-minute meeting. It is evident in how I approach the family. If you say, "Hi, it's nice to meet you" and shake hands and introduce yourself, you are showing respect.

Response of Nurse Heather Hart, who works with dying patients:

In palliative care, I don't know from one day to the next if the patient I've got is still going to be there the next time I'm back at work. Some patients are only there for a very short period of time. So it is really important to be able to quickly establish a collaborative relationship with the person because this may be your one and only chance. For example, one day I worked with a young woman with very advanced cancer. I had never in my life seen anyone so completely emaciated. There was something about this woman—an incredible spirit. I was caring for her during the morning, and close to noon I just spontaneously said, "You know, you have such an incredible spirit about you." At the same time I said this, I was also thinking, "How ironic that this tired flesh exudes such warmth and such a spirit." So she, with difficulty, went over to her desk and pulled out a sealed envelope. She showed me a picture of her that had been taken ten months earlier. She was a voluptuous, curvy woman in a bathing suit, smiling on vacation. That was her way of saying, "This is who I am." The spirit that I had observed was captured in the photo.

This was our starting point for talking about the many changes she had experienced. The biggest change was the incredible change in her physical appearance. I quickly learned from this discussion that her goal was not to become bitter. She said, "I don't want to become bitter about this, I want to stay who I am, maintain that spirit, the essence of who I am despite what you see on the outside." I had just met this woman when this encounter occurred but because I was able to get to know this woman and her goals quickly, our collaborative relationship continued for a couple of weeks. I think collaboration can happen in a very short time. You need to be present in that moment, and pick up cues from the person that indicate that it is going to be okay to venture into this topic with them.

The nurses concur that a collaborative partnership approach can be used in brief encounters. Nurse Irene Leboeuf's response reflects the particular importance of the nurse's language and nonverbal behaviour in brief collaborative nurse-person encounters. As explained in Chapter 5, the language that health professionals use and the way that they speak to people convey important messages about the balance of power between professionals and patients.

Nurse Heather Hart's example underscores the fact that a collaborative partnership is possible even after knowing a person for a short time. Nonetheless, the nurse needs to be skilled enough to know what key questions to pose to quickly gather the relevant information within a relatively short period of time. One of the common misconceptions about a collaborative partnership is that it takes time to develop. The development of a collaborative partnership is definitely facilitated by having intimate knowledge of the other person and her situation. This knowledge can take time to acquire. When the nurse knows the person over a period of time and accompanies the person and her family through various life events and/or illness experiences, the nurse and the person get to know one another in ways that are different from that which occurs during brief, episodic encounters. Nonetheless, nurses often meet people during periods of change, crisis, and life transition and, during these times, people are usually more vulnerable and more open to forming relationships with nurses. This can certainly expedite the development of a collaborative partnership.

There are many aspects of time that will affect the behaviour of both the nurse and the person and, thus, the manner in which they will be able to collaborate. The amount of time available for nurse-person interactions will affect the collaborative partnership as discussed in Chapter 4.

Question 9: What are the advantages of collaborating with people over an extended period of time?

Response of Nurse Irene Leboeuf, who works with brain tumour patients:

One advantage is that a nurse working with a person in crisis can use her knowledge of the person that she has acquired during noncrises events in order to nurse them collaboratively during crisis. For example, I was nursing a patient who had surgery and during that experience I noticed that he was very persistent in getting his questions answered. Three months after the crisis was over, the patient and his family did not remember that he had this strength. I met with them and said, "I remember three months ago, when you had this experience, I noticed that Mr. Jones was very persistent. When you're going through a challenging time, sometimes we forget that we have these tools. Perhaps you might be able to use some of this persistence now?" When you're working with people in the short-term, it's more difficult to have this knowledge.

Response of Nurse Diane Lowden, who works with patients with multiple sclerosis (MS):

I work with a population of patients who we follow over a very long period of time. I've been working at the MS clinic now for six years and am still working with people I met the first week I was here. I try to meet people at their first visit to the clinic. This helps shape their expectation of what is offered through our clinic, what some of the issues are that we can deal with together, and how we will work together. I work to help people be aware of how they might use me over time. I give them some suggestions as to the kinds of things we might work on. I think that setting the stage very early in your relationship with people that you will be working with over this long illness trajectory is useful. We determine together at which points in time it might be useful to have contact. I think setting some of that groundwork very early on facilitates collaboration over time.

One advantage of working with people over such a long time is that I get to know them well: what their everyday lives are like, their values and beliefs, what is meaningful, who their resources are, their personal strengths, and ways of reacting and coping with everyday and stressful events. This type of in-depth information and understanding of people can only develop with time and across different circumstances. Although there are definite advantages for collaboration of getting to know people over time, in some situations due to the nature of the experience it is possible to "bypass" the usual time required to gain in-depth knowledge of the person. This requires astute observation skills, sensitivity, excellent communication skills, and exquisite timing to get a sense of the essence of the person in a short time frame.

It takes time to develop a collaborative partnership. Working with people over time, the nurse acquires intimate knowledge of the person that can greatly facilitate collaborative partnership. The first phase of the process of collaborative partnership that we described in Chapter 3 was "getting to know the person." The more the nurse knows the person, the more the relationship can gain in strength and depth, and this can readily facilitate the remaining phases of the collaborative partnership. When the nurse knows the person over a period of time and accompanies the person and his family through various life events and/or illness experiences, the nurse and the person get to know one another in ways that are different from those experienced during brief, episodic encounters.

The timing of nurse-person encounters should also be considered in collaborative partnership. Nurses often meet people during periods of change, crisis, and life transition. During these events, people are usually more vulnerable and more open to forming relationships with nurses and other helping professionals. This can certainly expedite the development of a collaborative partnership.

The significance of first encounters is going to be very different if that first encounter is going to be the only encounter with the person, compared to if that first encounter is the first of many encounters that will take place over time. If the first encounter is the first of many, then the nurse uses this first meeting as an opportunity to set the stage for subsequent encounters. A group of Swedish researchers explored public health nurses' perceptions of the first encounter between nurses and parents of newborns. They found that nurses viewed the first home visit encounter as being critical for setting the tone for future encounters and they emphasized the importance of playing down the nurse's professional status so that the encounter was between two people (Jansson et al.,

2001). If the first encounter is the only encounter, then the nurse needs to be, as Nurse Diane Lowden remarks, very astute and skilled in setting the tone and the conditions for that one encounter.

Some of the strategies that we described in Chapter 5 are useful early in the relationship for laying the groundwork. For example, in Chapter 5 we discussed the value of explicitly discussing with the person his expectations for collaboration, the benefits of this approach, and the role that each partner can play.

Yet another aspect of time concerns where people are with respect to their illness experience. When people are acutely ill their ability to collaborate may be hampered temporarily. The nurse can work collaboratively with people who are acutely ill or in crisis, but the form that collaboration takes may differ in these circumstances. The nurse continuously assesses the degree of collaboration that can be expected of the person and modifies his approach based on this assessment. During times of acute illness or crisis, nurses often need to take the lead and may be more directive because that's what the situation calls for. In situations where the nurse assesses that the person is unable to collaborate (i.e., acutely ill or in crisis), then the nurse does most of the work. However, this does not mean that the nurse cannot continue to work with the person's goals or incorporate the person's perspective into his care plan. As people recover or the crisis subsides, the nurse's role should change to encourage greater participation by the person. The nurse might still play a very active role and coach the person on how to assume greater responsibility.

CONCLUSION

In Chapter 4 we identified some of the factors that shape collaborative partnership. In this chapter, we have revisited some of the factors that nurses find particularly challenging in practicing within a collaborative partnership approach. Our clinical experts, drawing from their knowledge and experience, have shared their interesting insights concerning how they have dealt with these challenges. Although the partner's culture, gender, beliefs, language, and communication skills are challenges to collaborative partnership, these challenges need to be understood and recognized as surmountable.

The challenges explored underscore the complexity of collaborative partnership. One of the emerging trends in health care delivery research is to understand the effects of culture and gender on health and health care. Few have examined what the effects are of these factors on collaborative partnership, but it seems likely that these factors do play a role, and warrant further study.

Context, time, and timing affect the collaborative partnership. Hospital, clinic, home, and other settings present their own unique set of challenges. Nurses need to be aware of the physical, environmental and organizational features of a particular setting to determine how the setting is affecting collaborative partnership.

Some setting factors are more easily modifiable than others. It is those factors that are under the nurse's control that should be the focus of the nurse's efforts.

KEY TERMS

constructivism	**enculturation**
cultural awareness	**ethnocentrism**
cultural knowledge	

SUGGESTED READINGS

Cioffi, J. (2003). Communicating with culturally and linguistically diverse patients in an acute care setting: Nurses' experiences. *International Journal of Nursing Studies, 40,* 299-306. A study that examines nurses' experiences in working with culturally and linguistically diverse patients.

Jansson, A., Petersson, K., & Uden, G. (2001). Nurses' first encounters with parents of newborn children—Public health nurses' views of a good meeting. *Journal of Clinical Nursing, 10,* 140-151. A study that shows how setting influences the nurse-person relationship and the balance of power.

Street, R. L. (2002). Gender differences in health care provider-patient communication: Are they due to style, stereotypes, or accommodation? *Patient Education and Counseling, 48,* 201-206. This article describes the literature on gender differences in health care provider-patient communication.

Chapter 8

ASK THE EXPERTS II: COLLABORATION AND THE NURSE-PERSON RELATIONSHIP

I believe there are many ways to navigate any illness experience. . . . I am curious and open to their experience and want to understand about it from them. . . . The experience is theirs and how they deal with it is also theirs.
—Nurse Gillian Taylor

After reading this chapter you should be able to:
- Describe some of the challenges that are common to any helping relationship and how these play out in a collaborative partnership relationship
- Identify different ways of approaching some of these challenges in your practice

In this chapter, our panel of experts addresses challenges related to the nurse-person relationship and offers some specific suggestions on ways to deal with these challenges. We address challenges such as how nurses can collaborate when people have different expectations for their relationship with the nurse, the role each will play, and the nurse's experience and background. Another challenge concerns the boundaries of professional partnership and other forms of partnership, such as friendship. The different forms and variations on collaborative partnership are also discussed when we address issues of personal safety and communication modality.

We also explore the nature of the ending of collaborative partnerships. Although we described the process of collaborative partnership in Chapter 3, we did not include an examination of how a collaborative partnership ends. In addition, we explore the limitations and benefits of collaborative partnerships from the perspective of our clinical experts.

Question 1: Some people believe professionals are the "experts" who know what is best. Can a nurse use a collaborative partnership approach with people who hold this belief?

Response of Nurse Cindy Dalton, who works in the community:

People who see the health professional as the expert may expect the nurse to take more of the initiative or assume more control for directing both the interaction and the person's care. However, people can learn to collaborate with you, and you can teach them to collaborate. Collaboration does not look the same with everybody. To collaborate, the nurse needs to shape the collaborative partnership process to the person's ability. You will play less of a leading role with someone who wants to be in charge of his or her care or with someone who has good problem-solving abilities. On the other hand, you might be more directive with people who expect you to give them expert advice. However, you are always working towards shifting power from the nurse to the person. In each encounter you look for opportunities to give the person more power.

In the beginning, when working with people who see the professional as an expert, it is important for the nurse to take on that role as expert. Usually these people ask a lot of questions. When they ask good questions, you can tell them that their questions are good. This helps to build their confidence in their ability to participate in their care. Eventually as the type of questions or the nature of the questions they pose changes over time, you can point out to them that they have mastered a topic. In this way, you enhance their awareness of their own ability to learn and master information or skills.

Some people have difficulty acknowledging that they are learning and becoming more knowledgeable, and they may tell you that they still need you and your expert knowledge. In such cases, I reassure them that I am not going to leave them on their own, even once they feel that they have acquired the expertise. However, if your assessment reveals that they are doing really well, that they have knowledge and are able to problem solve effectively on their own, then you should point this out to them. You can give them specific, concrete examples of what they know and how they have effectively managed different situations. You can consistently highlight their expertise. Eventually with this repeated feedback, many people gain confidence in their own knowledge and abilities and begin to work more as partners in their care.

Response of Nurse Diane Lowden, who works with patients with multiple sclerosis:

Some people are very motivated to enter into a collaborative partnership relationship. They really want to work with health professionals in this way and are capable of doing so. They engage very readily in the collaborative process and the exploration that is part of this approach. For other people, this is a new idea and they find such an approach a bit foreign. When you ask exploratory questions (for example, "Tell me about . . ." or "How would you approach that problem") and try to set the stage for a collaborative partnership relationship, they are not sure how to respond. They are perhaps accustomed to medical encounters where the health professional tells them what to do. For these people, this idea of collaboration may be a very new idea that may take a little time for them to understand and accept. But it can certainly be done.

Response of Nurse Deborah Moudarres, who works with people who are mentally ill:

Some people are challenging to collaborate with because they may expect the nurse to take over and solve their problems. If I used a traditional hierarchical "nurse-as-expert" approach then I would tell them, "This is what you need to do. Try this and off you go." Instead, I want to engage people in exploring and finding out what it is they need and want and how they want to do it. In the first few contacts with anyone, it is important to explain what my expertise is and what expertise the person brings to our work together. This is particularly important when working with people who view professionals as the experts. I explain that I am the expert at helping them to identify and explore their concerns and at facilitating their problem solving. I also explain that I have knowledge about how people cope with and adjust to illness and other life transitions. At the same time, I highlight they are the only ones who know what their situation means to them, how it affects their life, and what may work best for them.

Sometimes people say to me "What do you think I should do?" In these situations I tell people that I have found that it is often not helpful for me to tell people what to do. I explain that everyone is unique and, therefore, it is important for people to find ways that will work for them. What I think might be helpful may not work for them. I encourage people to come up with their own ideas whenever possible. So I usually reflect the question back to them. I might say, "What is it that you want?" It is only after exhausting attempts to have the person come up with their own ideas as to what they might do or try that I offer suggestions. Even when I do offer suggestions, I always explain that my suggestions may or may not work and we discuss how they might want to modify my suggestion to best fit their situation. After awhile of working in this way, some people come to realize that they play a key role in this collaborative problem-solving process, and they are surprised at how active a role they can play. Other people comment on how much work this can be. However, when they experience success and are able to reach a goal, they feel extremely gratified and motivated because they themselves have brought about the changes they are experiencing.

Response of Nurse Gillian Taylor, who works with children who have arthritis:

In some cultures, professionals are held in high esteem. They tend to be viewed as experts who hold the answers and solutions to every problem and situation. Given that professionals are viewed in this way, some people expect and want the professional to make all the decisions about their care. To ask people from these cultures to collaborate and be active participants in their care can be stressful and may actually undermine their opinion of you as a professional.

Response of Nurse Heather Hart, who works in palliative care:

In some situations the nurse needs to be more directive and assume the lead, usually in response to a person's or family's needs or at their request. For example, in my practice in palliative care many families haven't been through a death before.

It's a new experience, and so they may want me to be quite directive as to what they might do at that time. I still think that I have a collaborative partnership relationship with them though, if underlying this period of greater nurse directiveness, there is a relationship based on respect and reciprocity. The scale may tip a little, so that I am assuming more of the lead in decision making, but the balance of power is just shifted a little for the moment.

Earlier, in Chapter 4, we discussed the factors that shape collaborative partnership. The beliefs of both the person and the nurse were very influential factors. People's beliefs and expectations about how they will relate to health care professionals are in large part culturally determined. These beliefs may also reflect generational effects because some studies have found that older people are less likely to want to share in care decision making with health professionals (Sainio & Lauri, 2003; Thompson, Pitts, & Schwankovsky, 1993). The bottom line is that each person needs to be seen as an individual. How one person will prefer to and be able to collaborate is different from another person. There are different forms or levels of collaboration, and the nurse should tailor the collaborative partnership to fit the individual person, their preferences, and their ability to play a role in their care at different times (Roberts, 2002). Our clinical experts suggest that the nurse should work with the person in the way the person prefers, but nonetheless the nurse aims to shift the balance of power to the person whenever appropriate.

The other idea that follows from this is that people can learn to collaborate with the nurse. Nurse Cindy Dalton described how the nurse can help people learn to play a more active role in their care. Although some people may at first prefer to be submissive and adopt a "good" or "compliant" patient role (Cahill, 1998), they may in fact be interested in learning more about how to be a partner in their care. Others may believe that they are expected to be submissive—and will therefore leave the decision making to the professional (Henderson, 2002). People who have never experienced a partnership with a health professional may not even be aware that this could be possible, and other people may be fearful of playing a role in decision making because they have no previous experience. To help people learn how to collaborate, the nurse may need to carefully assess which of the nurse, person, nurse-person relationship, or environmental factors (as described in Chapter 4) are operating in this situation, and which could be modified to encourage the person to become a more active partner.

Nurse Deborah Moudarres highlighted some valuable strategies that may help a person learn to work in a collaborative partnership with a nurse. First, she discussed the importance of the nurse setting the stage for a collaborative partnership in the first encounters between the nurse and person. Nurse Moudarres also explained how discussing what expertise the person and the nurse bring to their relationship is also a useful strategy to promote the person's involvement in her care and in the collaborative partnership.

Question 2: Some people believe that the professional has to experience a situation personally to be credible. How can a nurse work collaboratively with people who feel this way?

Response of Nurse Cindy Dalton, who works in the community:

I have dealt with this often in my practice. While working in community health, I visited postpartum mothers in their homes. One day, I arranged to see a mother who had just given birth to her first child. On the telephone, she told me that she really wanted to breast-feed but that it was not going well. I arrived at the mother's home and we began to discuss how things were going. Then the doorbell rang. Ten women were at the door. The mother let them into the apartment, and they sat down and joined us. I did not understand what was happening. So I asked the mother if she wished to continue our visit or whether I should come back at a more convenient time. She explained that her friends had come because they knew I was coming and they wanted to be present. She explained that her friends were mothers who had breast-fed and that they had some questions they wanted to ask me. I agreed to respond to their questions. They wanted to know: Did I have personal experience breast-feeding? What were my beliefs and values about breast-feeding? What did I know about it? These ten women had come to check out my expertise! They admitted that they had come because they had been trying to help their friend establish breast-feeding and feared that I would discourage breast-feeding.

I acknowledged that her friends were all experts in breast-feeding, and noted how lucky she was to have their support and expertise. I explained that I was not a mother, so I did not have firsthand experience. However, I did have several years of experience doing postpartum visits and had acquired knowledge from the women I had nursed. I told them that I thought breast-feeding was best for the baby's health. My goal was to help their friend successfully breast-feed because that is what their friend told me she wanted. I suggested to the new mother that we discuss this together and come up with some ideas that might be useful to her. There are many ways of acquiring expert knowledge and it does not have to be through firsthand personal experience.

Response of Nurse Gillian Taylor, who works with children who have arthritis:

Early in my career, parents would frequently say to me, "How could you know about that?" or "You can't possibly know what we are going through." Now, I can't remember when I was last asked such questions. I suspect that these types of questions come up when you offer advice that doesn't really fit the people or their situation. So if that type of question does arise, then the nurse should inquire, "Is there anything that I have said or done today or in the past that indicates that I am not listening to you?"

Nurses who have clinical experience can say to families, "I am a nurse who has worked with many families whose child has X. I try to listen and learn from families about what helps and what doesn't." Families want to hear that you know how to help them deal with their issues. This is very reassuring to them. Less experienced nurses or students can read descriptive, qualitative studies that describe patients' and families' experiences and then say to the family, "I've read something recently about (and tell what you have read); does this speak to you?"

When parents are frustrated with me or with the health care team because they feel that we have no idea what they are going through, I will then say, "I don't know what you are going through. But I have sat with other families who have had a similar experience and I have learned to appreciate how frightening this is, and I want to understand your experience." What I have to offer is respect for, rather than firsthand knowledge of, the specific experience.

I believe there are many ways to navigate any illness experience. When I share this belief with families I find that they are reassured. I try to share with them that I am curious and open to their experience and want to understand about it from them. What is most important is to validate patients' and families' feelings and experiences and to communicate that you have listened. The experience is theirs and how they deal with it is also theirs. One mother recently told me, "Nobody really understood, but you always listened. You never made me feel bad about it. You let me handle it."

I think there is an advantage on some levels of not having personally experienced what your patients are going through. When you have personally gone through a similar experience there may be a danger of seeing it through your own eyes rather than through their eyes. It may narrow what you attend to, as there may be a tendency to attend to information that validates your own experience. Parents do ask me about issues that I do have personal experience with, such as child discipline. They may ask, "Do you have children? What did you do?" I will admit that I have a child. But I will refer to what the literature or other parents have found useful.

Sometimes when people question nurses' credibility they are responding to the nurse's devaluing of their expertise and knowledge. People who live with chronic illness and their family and caregivers often become very skilled in illness management and develop in-depth knowledge of the illness. Patients and caregivers have reported feeling that health care professionals often fail to recognize their expertise or feel threatened by it (Allen, 2000; Thorne, Nyhlin, & Paterson, 2000). Also, when people feel vulnerable and are afraid, they need to feel that they are being heard. Once they feel that the nurse has understood their perception of their experience, then they are less concerned about whether the nurse has had the same experience.

Nurses use many different types of knowledge in their practice. They use scientific knowledge or empirical knowledge, ethical knowledge, aesthetic knowledge (i.e., knowledge of what to do and how to do it) and personal knowledge (knowledge of oneself and knowing how one comes across in interpersonal interactions) (Carper, 1978; Chinn & Kramer, 2004). If the nurse has not had a firsthand personal experience with an event it does not mean that the nurse cannot appreciate that experience. The nurse can draw on many different ways of knowing, not just personal experience. Nurses accumulate knowledge and experience through practice that gives them credibility and communicates competency. The clinical experts note that they may or may not have had the same personal experience as the person, but they do have professional experience helping people deal with that particular experience. It is this professional experience that nurses often draw on.

Question 3: In a collaborative partnership, how much should the nurse disclose about herself?

Response of Nurse Heather Hart, who works in palliative care:

The short answer to your question about how much should the nurse disclose about herself is "yes." From the start when you meet someone you should be disclosing information about your professional background and experience, particularly experience related to the patient's own health or illness experience. For example, when I worked with MS (multiple sclerosis) patients it was important for them to know that I had previous experience nursing people with MS. This information gives the patient and the family some notion of where you are coming from and it provides you with some credibility.

I think that it is also appropriate at times to disclose personal information. The decision to share personal information with the patient and the family is done selectively and deliberately. What to disclose and when to disclose it is determined by the nurse. Information is shared with a particular goal in mind. One important outcome of sharing personal information with people is that it builds a sense of reciprocity into the relationship. Reciprocity is important in a relationship. There is a give and take in the relationship. If the family shares personal information with me, I share some with them.

Selectively sharing personal information can also facilitate engagement. A bit of disclosure is almost a natural progression in a collaborative partnership that goes on over time. People are naturally curious about basic personal information, and most people do ask these types of questions at some time. Questions such as "How long have you worked here?" "Are you married?" and "Do you have children?" are common. I have no problem answering these questions. In my experience, an outcome of disclosing this basic personal information is that people learn a bit more about you. Disclosure can be a useful tool to help people get involved with you and stay involved in a relationship with you. People get to know you better and in a different way. You are not a stranger any longer, but a real person with a story. It also is a way of equalizing power in the relationship.

When people learn that you have had life experiences and seen difficult things before, this tells them that you can handle or cope with whatever they may bring to you. When I was a graduate student working with MS patients and their families, people saw me as a student. In some situations they sought to protect you from their issues because they saw students as inexperienced and young. Families would ask me questions about my education and personal background. When I responded to these questions they learned that I was not as young as they thought. The quality of the relationship always changed after this disclosure. In fact, one woman told me that she had a whole new respect for me because I had "lived."

I was visiting a couple in their home. In one meeting we discussed at length how the patient's disease impacted their relationship as a couple. The discussion was a painful one for the couple, because each partner shared many uncomfortable feelings. At the end of the visit, they said to me, "Now it is our turn." They wanted to ask me some questions about my personal relationships. They asked if I was involved in a relationship and for how long. I answered these simple questions with short answers, but did not go into details. The couple was satisfied with the basic information that I gave them and asked no further questions. This disclosure injected a bit of balance into that collaborative encounter. I answered their questions to show that I too was part of a couple and knew about the complexities of couple relationships.

Selectively disclosing personal information for a specific purpose is not the same thing as "unloading your personal baggage." That is never appropriate. Sharing personal information is not a social thing, but is a deliberate action whose purpose is professional not personal.

Response of Nurse Gillian Taylor, who works with children who have arthritis:

Disclosure is a tricky thing. The nurse needs to understand why she is disclosing personal information. When the nurse discloses her own experience it can burden the patient and family. Patient and families are going through their own experience and they don't need to hear the nurse's personal story, particularly if the nurse's experience is really devastating, such as in the case of a death.

Often nurses share their own personal stories to show the family that they understand what the family is going through. A danger is that when the nurse discloses personal information she may in effect minimize the family's experiences and may take away from the uniqueness of their personal experience. I think that can backfire because we are most helpful when we appreciate the family's unique experience. What to disclose and how much to disclose depends on the timing of disclosure, whether the nurse has had the experience, the nature of the experience, and what purpose the disclosure serves.

Sometimes, patients will share with us an event that has caused them great embarrassment such as when a child throws a temper tantrum in the middle of the grocery aisle. I might empathize with their experience by sharing with them what I felt when my daughter had one of her temper tantrums. I might tell them that "I wanted to slink out of there unnoticed." This is a way of normalizing the experience and the feelings for them. In such a situation, disclosing my own experience helps to communicate an understanding of their discomfort and may help to strengthen the nurse-patient/family relationship. It may also help the patients to deal with the emotion accompanying the event and allow them to move on to dealing with the event.

I can also see how revealing personal information may be used to communicate hope to the patient and family. One nurse told a young 16-year-old girl who had just undergone hip replacement that another staff nurse had also had a hip replacement. The other nurse then visited the patient, and they immediately connected.

It is important for the nurse first to ask herself some reflective questions, such as "Why am I telling someone this?" "What benefit will come from sharing this information?" The nurse shares personal information to connect with patients, not to be their friend. Remaining neutral and providing a place to come to share information in a safe, comfortable environment are often what the patient needs.

Response of Nurse Jackie Townshend, who works with children with cystic fibrosis:

Disclosure is a delicate issue. Over time and with experience I think you become more comfortable about disclosing. Early in your career, many nurses believe that being professional means not disclosing and that personal information only goes one way. But there are times when sharing information about yourself is appropriate and useful. A collaborative partnership requires a nonhierarchical stance. Sharing a little something about yourself gives a counterbalance to the relationship. If the patients are the only ones doing any disclosing, it is a bit of a one-sided relationship. When you disclose something, it balances things.

I am thinking of one recent example from my practice. I recently ended my work with a 12-year-old boy who I had nursed since he was 4 years old. We had a strong attachment and the ending process was difficult for both of us. He felt that I was abandoning him and his family. I shared with him my own feelings of sadness and pain. I described to him some of the other goodbyes in my own life and used these examples to illustrate how ending can be positive. I could have used examples from other patients, but it was more powerful to use examples from my own experience. He needed to see that even if people care they sometimes have to say goodbye. As I was disclosing my own personal feelings in this situation, I was fully aware that the reason for my disclosure was to help the boy. This is really the best indicator of when it is appropriate to disclose personal information about yourself. My disclosure helped him be able to share his own feelings.

A study by McCann and Baker (2001) found that mental health patients and their families felt that disclosure by the nurse put them at ease, narrowed the power gap between themselves and the nurse, and helped them find areas of common interest with the nurse. They perceived that disclosure promoted the development of the nurse-person relationship and had therapeutic value.

Our experts agree that disclosure of personal information is a useful strategy that nurses have at their disposal. Nonetheless, they caution that this strategy needs to be used carefully. Disclosing personal information conveys openness, and openness is an essential ingredient of a collaborative partnership. The nurse needs to strike a delicate balance between having a professional relationship with the person and having a friendship. Some personal disclosures may shift the relationship from a professional helping relationship to a friendship, thus upsetting the delicate balance of collaborative partnership. On the other hand, some personal disclosures may serve to deepen the level of intimacy within the professional relationship.

The nurse has to consider the purpose of the disclosure and what effects sharing personal information might have on the person. If the purpose of the disclosure is to connect with or find common ground with the person, then disclosure may be beneficial. If, on the other hand, the nurse's disclosure burdens the person by putting the person in the role of counselor or friend, then disclosure may have a deleterious effect. What further differentiates a personal disclosure that is therapeutic from one that could be harmful is the timing of when the disclosure is made.

Question 4: Are there situations in which the nurse is more directive and assumes more of the lead or in which collaboration is not appropriate?

Response of Nurse Lucia Fabijan, who works with people who are mentally ill:

I think there are situations where the nurse is directive, but I would still consider that I was using a collaborative partnership approach if the person wants or requires this approach. Of course, I would hope that we could develop to the point at which that may no longer be necessary. In our mental health setting, if someone is acutely psychotic there will be instances where you certainly cannot collaborate. It's crisis intervention. The patient may be saying, "I'm fine, I'm fine, I'm fine," and you are saying, "No, you are not. We need to get you help and we're going to walk over to the emergency room." Another situation that calls for the nurse to take charge is when you are working with a family with issues related to violence.

Response of Nurse Jackie Townshend, who works with children with cystic fibrosis:

A tough situation in pediatrics is when we need to call in Youth Protection. Those are difficult moments and sometimes you can maintain a collaborative partnership practice throughout that type of situation, and sometimes it can destroy a relationship depending on the outcomes.

Response of Nurse Deborah Moudarres, who works with people who are mentally ill:

In some special situations and circumstances, it is not that you are being noncollaborative—I never think "We're no longer going to collaborate." For example, there have been a few difficult situations where I've actually had to call the police because I have assessed the situation and feel that the person may be a threat to themselves or to others. At that point, I have to take charge. I think it's very difficult for a nurse who is using a collaborative partnership approach to get to the point where you have to do something like that. I still feel I'm collaborating because I think that our overall goal that we agreed to was that we would work in a therapeutic relationship together.

This is a health-promoting interaction, so the goal is for the person to be well. At that moment they may not agree with me because they have abandoned some of their goals. At those times, collaboration does look a little different. Usually I've found that you can come back to an understanding that you're working in the same direction.

Response of Nurse Diane Lowden, who works with patients with multiple sclerosis:

When patient safety is at issue, the nurse needs to be directive. I remember working with one couple and the nature of their relationship was unclear. The team felt that the patient's partner was making decisions that were not in her best interests and were in fact risky for her. We tried to explore with the partner his understanding of her situation and the rationale behind his decisions. However at the end, dissatisfied with his answers, the team became much more directive. The team told him, "You need to know that if you make this decision, that this is going against medical advice." It was a patient safety issue that precipitated this directive approach because the collaborative partnership approach just didn't seem to be working and we were concerned about the risks to the patient's health in that situation.

All of our clinical experts agree that collaborative partnership takes a different form when the person's safety is an issue or when law requires nurses to act (i.e., reporting child abuse). Partnership may also be more limited in crises or emergency situations or when the person's judgment is impaired. The nurse can continue to work collaboratively at some level in some situations by working with the person's broader goals. For example, a common situation that often arises with elderly people is that they are no longer able to live at home safely and yet are not able to recognize this. The nurse may work collaboratively to help the person reach his or her broader goal of maintaining independence, but within an environment that is safe. The nurse would not necessarily support the elderly person's desire to remain in the home but may explore choices of alternative housing. In other instances, the nurse no longer collaborates with the person whose safety is at stake, but rather collaborates with the person's family or significant others.

Question 5: Nursing in a community setting or an ambulatory care setting often involves telephone contact with people. Is it possible to use a collaborative partnership approach during telephone contact or is face-to-face contact with people necessary?

Response of Nurse Diane Lowden, who works with patients with multiple sclerosis:

The telephone is a tool that I use extensively with the population that I work with, because some people with MS have a significant amount of disability that makes it difficult for them to come to hospital. In my experience a lot of therapeutic nursing work can be provided by telephone. I find that if I have met with somebody previously face-to-face, then the phone is a useful tool that can extend our work beyond face-to-face encounters. The interactions are actually quite similar.

However, I do find that the reverse is much more difficult. If I have not met the person face-to-face nor done a nursing assessment, but I have had telephone conversations with them because they have called repeatedly with questions about their care or symptoms, then I find it is difficult to situate or understand the context of the telephone contacts. It is difficult for me to understand how all these bits and pieces of information that are acquired in telephone contacts fit together. In these cases, I will say to the person, "We've never actually met and I think it would be important for us to do that. We've talked about your bladder infections and your medication tolerance. There are a lot of pieces that are missing for me here, and I really would like to understand a little bit more about you and your family and what some of the issues are that we're dealing with so I can work with you most effectively."

Response of Nurse Jackie Townshend, who works with children with cystic fibrosis (CF):

I have had a lot of phone contact with patients and their families in my practice with families who have a child with CF. Parents call all the time. Collaboration is really a way of being, so it can be used anywhere and in any setting. However, there are some special challenges to collaboration on the phone. The biggest challenge is that you cannot observe nonverbal behaviour, so you are missing some potentially important information. For this reason, it might be easier to use a collaborative partnership approach when working with people over the telephone if you know the person or family well. Your in-depth knowledge of them makes it easier to collaborate effectively without the nonverbal cues. I find working collaboratively over the telephone is difficult when I do not know the person. Knowing people, knowing how they will react to what you will say, and how to say what you want to say helps you to be effective in collaborating on the phone.

As Nurse Jackie Townshend stated, collaborative partnership is a way of *being*, thus it can be used in many different contexts. Telephone contact has been used in many different ways in nursing practice. It has been used to provide support, to follow up on health concerns between face-to-face contacts, to do teaching, and to provide grief counseling (McBride & Rimer, 1999). Our experts note that there are special challenges when using the telephone as a means of communication in a collaborative partnership. In Chapter 4, we described how the communication and interpersonal skills of both the nurse and the person can influence the nature of the collaborative partnership. For some nurses and for some people, the telephone can be an effective means of communication for maintaining a relationship. Others might find telephone contact difficult or intrusive. The lack of nonverbal cues may make it more difficult for the nurse to develop a collaborative partnership; however, this depends on the nurse's skill and the person's ease in communicating via telephone. Communicating via telephone may be easier once the nurse has gotten to know the person (i.e., moved beyond the "getting to know" phase described in Chapter 3).

Question 6: What does the process of ending or terminating a relationship look like in a collaborative partnership? Is it different than in a noncollaborative approach?

Response of Nurse Cindy Dalton, who works in the community:

The key difference in ending a collaborative partnership relationship versus a more traditional hierarchical relationship is how the ending takes place. When you nurse with a collaborative partnership approach, you invite the person to participate in a discussion of termination. The person should be involved to the greatest extent possible in deciding if, when, and how the relationship will end, as well as deciding who will remain involved or who might get involved when the active relationship with the nurse ends.

In some cases, the decision to terminate is made jointly. I might see that the relationship could end because we have accomplished our goals or my assistance is no longer needed. I might then be the one to broach the subject of ending our work. I would explain to the person what it is that I had observed that made me think that this might be the time to end our relationship. Then I would ask the person what it would be like for them if we were to discuss ending. Sometimes people have already thought about this themselves, but have not mentioned this to me. These people are ready to discuss ending. At other times, people have not yet considered ending the relationship, but they are open to discussing this when you introduce the topic. In other cases, the person initiates this discussion. The person may feel that he has achieved his goals or perhaps he is ready to continue on his own.

Even if termination is nurse initiated and must happen without consulting the person (such as when the nurse is leaving her position), the person can still share in deciding how the termination will take place. This should be negotiated with the person to best meet his needs.

As with ending any relationship, it is important to set aside time to talk about the impact of the ending on the person. When you are terminating a collaborative partnership, you are saying goodbye not only to the work that you have done together, but also to the relationship. Thus, the relationship is very much at the forefront of your discussion. At termination, the nurse and person review the highlights of their work together, their goals and achievements. You consider: Where was the person when we began? How far has she come? Where is she heading? How much work is still to be done? What can the person do on her own? What, if anything, does she need other professionals or resources to help her with? You take some time to review the important points of your work together, that is, those points where change took place, learning occurred, or the person's involvement in the her own care increased.

With some people, especially those who are less confident in their abilities or who view professionals as experts, you need to reassure them that they are ready to deal with things on their own. You can reframe the ending; that is, you can help them view the ending in a positive light. You can explain to them that it is not so much an ending, but the beginning of a new phase in their experience.

Ending a collaborative relationship means that the door is often not completely closed. The person may be referred to someone or someplace else, but often you let the person know he can come back. You can negotiate clear guidelines with him for how and when this might be needed, so he will know how to make this decision.

Response of Nurse Margaret Eades, who works with patients with cancer:

The initiation and termination of a relationship often vary depending on the nature of the work that patients and their families identify as needing to be done. In my work as a clinical nurse specialist in oncology, the idea of initiating or terminating a relationship has less meaning with other patient populations because of the unpredictability of cancer.

I prefer the word transition because it reflects more accurately the nature of the work. I transition in and out of different issues that we may be working on together but I don't terminate the relationship. The relationship may continue for several years. I see people and their families over many years, as they come in and out of the health care system or when they have particular experiences, both expected and unexpected.

Let me tell you about a patient and family I was dealing with. A husband and wife identified that their family was in crisis and they wanted some help. Each of the family members had his or her own sets of concerns relative to the patient's illness and the extent of the illness. The husband's lymphoma was in an advanced stage and he needed to make decisions about a very aggressive treatment. He needed to know that this was going to be effective and that it would start soon because he could visibly see the progression of the tumour.

Meanwhile, the wife as the major caregiver was concerned about his well-being and supporting him. She was also concerned about the youngest daughter who was having difficulty coping with the fact that her father might die. In addition, the wife also needed to learn how to manage the family finances. She was supporting her elderly mother and a brother who was also newly diagnosed with an equally devastating disease. I spent time helping them articulate what the issues were, and to devise a plan to address their concerns. I was very involved with the family through the ups and downs of their experience until the husband's death. I went to the funeral and I am still involved with the wife and daughter. The notion of termination is incongruent with this type of nursing. I do terminate when someone lives out of town or when the patient dies, but I always leave the door open. A better term to describe the ending of a relationship is that it slowly fades away rather than ending.

Response of Nurse Deborah Moudarres, who works with people with mental illness:

When the nurse operates within a traditional hierarchical approach, it is often he or she who decides when the goals have been achieved and the relationship ends. This can happen whether the person agrees or not. Many nurses who use a professional-as-expert model (i.e., the traditional hierarchical model) in their practices end relationships with people because they fear dependency. In contrast, for nurses who use a collaborative partnership approach, termination involves mutual discussion and agreement between the person and the nurse. This is the ideal that you work toward and that actually occurs in most situations.

The ending of a collaborative relationship can be initiated by the person or by the nurse. Regular review of progress towards achieving goals is important. It is the nurse's role to ensure that this evaluation takes place. In these reviews, we jointly evaluate how we are progressing. In the midst of these discussions, the idea of ending can be raised.

Most of the time, in a collaborative partnership relationship, it is the person who decides that it is time to end. Sometimes the person feels that she has gained knowledge and skill and feels ready to go ahead on her own. A decrease in the frequency of contact with you can be an indicator of this. At other times, people initiate termination because they feel they have accomplished their goals or because they feel that our relationship is not working.

If there comes a time in my work with someone when no new concerns or goals are coming forth, I may be the one to mention that termination might be indicated. If I introduce the idea and the person does do not agree that it is time to terminate, we might decrease the frequency of our contacts as a way of making a gradual transition towards termination in the future when the person is comfortable. If the person agrees that the time might be right to end our working relationship, then we will work towards that.

Whether the person or the nurse initiates it, termination is a process that usually occurs over time. A review of the relationship and our work is always a part of this process. We will review and discuss what we have done, what we have learned, the progress we have made, and what has gone well. I always give concrete examples to illustrate this because this helps the person make the link between the skills and competencies they have gained and the outcomes we have observed. Also we discuss anything that the person may be concerned about in relation to ending our partnership. Some people need reassurance that they are capable of coping on their own. Others need reassurance that they can come back to see me if they have difficulty. I will often tell people that they can telephone and tell me about their progress. This strategy really gives the person control over the ending of the collaborative partnership.

Occasionally the person might wish to end our relationship, but I do not agree that the time is right. You cannot force someone to continue to see you. In these situations, if you take the opportunity to revisit the nature of the relationship and your work together, you can get things back on track and avert termination. However, in other situations what the nurse has to offer may not meet the person's needs. In these cases, I then offer to link the person with other services. I also usually tell them that they can come back to see me if they reconsider their decision.

The clinical experts agree that the essential difference between ending a nurse-person relationship that is based on a collaborative partnership and a relationship that is not based on collaboration is how the ending of the nurse-person relationship is determined. In a collaborative partnership, the ending is mutually agreed on and negotiated. Collaborative partnership involves mutual decision making throughout the process. When and how the ending occurs is yet another decision that the nurse and person discuss together. In Chapter 3, we described how negotiation was a key subprocess of the collaborative partnership. Negotiation may be required when the nurse and person have different ideas about when and how to end their active work.

The clinical experts' responses underscore the idea that in a collaborative partnership the relationship is open, which means that although a certain active phase of the relationship may come to a natural end, the relationship may be ongoing. The nurse may move in and out over the course of the person's life. For example, at times of crisis the person may decide to reinitiate contact with the nurse should he or she feel that this is needed. This may characterize the nurse-person relationship, particularly when the person is dealing with a chronic condition with remissions and exacerbations.

Termination was originally conceptualized as the last phase of the nurse-patient relationship. The process was a very linear process, and termination was the end of this process. The collaborative partnership process described in Chapter 3 is a circular and fluid process, with a beginning but no specific termination phase. The process is much more open ended. This idea of an open ending was echoed in a study of psychiatric nurses' lived experiences of nurse-patient relationships (Walsh, 1997). Nurses perceived that the endings of their relationships with patients were not final and not neatly "signed off." Furthermore, endings continued to have an effect long after the relationship had ended.

Question 7: What are the limitations or disadvantages of using a collaborative partnership approach in your practice?

Response of Nurse Jane Chambers-Evans, who works with adults in intensive care:

One limitation of a collaborative partnership approach to practice is that it requires a significant investment in terms of energy and self. Some people are concerned about being involved in that way with families. Even when it is very much an automatic response or the way you practice, it still requires an investment. Thinking about an upcoming meeting, about what you think the family might bring up and what you think you might want to ask them, takes energy. The problem-solving activities and the flexibility required of the nurse can drain you emotionally and intellectually. It's the wonderful part about a collaborative partnership approach, but it is also the downside of it.

Sometimes we haven't built into our health care system the resources to help nurses deal with the demands of collaborative partnership work. A lot of my colleagues are sometimes tired and unable to function at a high level. I use a group of my peers for support. We meet every week, talk about what we're doing, and provide support and consultation to one another. Sometimes we bring clinical cases to the group to obtain feedback and ideas. In other settings, nurses meet in small groups every two weeks to consult with colleagues and a supervisor. They can bring clinical situations and broader issues to the group for discussion. It is helpful to have others that you can talk to about your practice and get another perspective or ideas about where to go next.

I think some people would say collaboration also requires a lot of time. Sometimes I find time is an issue. Although it may take time, ultimately I think you are being more effective.

Response of Nurse Margaret Eades, who works with patients with cancer:

A collaborative approach takes time, and sometimes that is in conflict with the demands of the health care system. However, the two are not incompatible. You have to be very creative in making opportunities to move people forward. In a way, the time in hospitals or clinics is so short that it needs to be focused, which takes some creativity. Patients may not be ready to address issues that they need to address, particularly care interventions such as how to care for their wounds or colostomies, getting out of bed, assuming more self-care, and/or addressing issues of pain management. To get patients ready to address these issues even though they might not be ready to do so requires creativity and time—yet it needs to be done.

Working effectively within a collaborative partnership means knowing the person well enough to be in tune with his needs and goals, understanding what the person is going through, experiencing his suffering and pain, and responding to his vulnerability. It is by being open to the person's experience and working with him that the nurse is in a position to work collaboratively. Collaborative partnership embodies caring. Without caring, one cannot form a collaborative partnership (although not all caring gives rise to collaborative partnership). Caring by its nature requires involvement and investment of self and time. However, it is this investment in people and relationships that allows one to connect and to experience satisfaction, joy, and fulfillment (Benner & Wrubel, 1989). Involvement and investment can be stressful and energy depleting as Nurse Chambers-Evans pointed out. It also can be energizing, because it is through collaborative partnerships that people assume responsibility for change and growth.

One self-protective strategy that nurses routinely use is to distance themselves from people and not get involved. This has sometimes been done under the guise of so-called professionalism or, as Benner and Wrubel (1989) described it, "controlled caring." Strategies that nurses use to distance themselves include trivializing distress, cutting people off from expressing their fear and pain, keeping busy, focusing on physical care or technical procedures, and seeing nursing as a job. When nurses adopt these self-protective strategies they also limit their investment in the relationship and their ability to be enriched by the relationship and the joy and satisfaction that derives from connecting with people at a deeper level.

Collaborative partnership involves an investment that can be exhausting. The way to deal with this challenge is to build in strategies and organizational supports that prevent burn-out. Nurses may need to learn how to take time out and to re-energize. Moreover, nursing administrators who want to promote collaborative practice need to provide a supportive milieu for nurses who are using a collaborative partnership approach in their practice. This may involve ongoing clinical advising, whereby nurses have a forum in which they can discuss their practice and obtain support and guidance (Feeley & Gerez-Lirette, 1992; Murphy, 1994).

Another limitation of a collaborative partnership approach that was not mentioned by the experts but has often been cited by others is that collaborative partnership fosters overreliance of the person on the nurse and, therefore, this approach to care is too costly to the health care system. This is not the case. Collaborative partnership is built on mutual understanding, respect, and trust and, as such, persons feel more connected to the nurse than they would in a more traditional hierarchical model of care. Some fear that these feelings of connectedness and familiarity with the nurse foster dependency. On the contrary, the collaborative relationship often leads people to feel secure because they have come to trust in themselves and the nurse. These feelings of security may help the person tap into his or her own strengths and draw on resources to meet life's challenges. As an outcome of working collaboratively with the nurse, some people acquire greater knowledge and a broader repertoire of skills, and they eventually become more self-reliant. Moreover, they depend less not only on the nurse but on health care professionals and use fewer health care services. For the past decade, the Systems-Linked Research Unit on Health and Social Service Utilization at McMaster University has been examining these very issues. A consistent finding across many of their studies of the needs of vulnerable populations is that people who get the right type of service use the health care system more appropriately and this translates into impressive savings in health care costs (Browne et al., 2001)."

Question 8: If you had two minutes to convince colleagues to adopt a collaborative partnership approach in their practice, what would you tell them?

Response of Nurse Jane Chambers-Evans, who works with adults in intensive care:

I think it's important to describe collaborative practice in terms of the outcomes in your own area, so that colleagues can relate to collaborative practice. For people working with me, I tell them that by working together with patients we avoid getting into problems with families. We avoid conflicts. We will be able to make decisions together and we will be able to have families understand what it is we're trying to accomplish with the patient. For colleagues to engage in collaborative relationship it's no different than for families. They have to see there is some reason to engage in that type of practice.

Response of Nurse Lucia Fabijan, who works with people who are mentally ill:

I would tell them that they may see less "resistance" to the recommended plan of action, that people may actually show up for some appointments. I would also tell them that problems with "noncompliance" are really due to a lack of collaboration. There are better ways to look at this issue of noncompliance. There are reasons that people refuse to take medications. If we collaborate and figure out together what's going on behind that, there might be a way in which to encourage people to take their medication for a period of time. So I often find I have to use key words like resistance and noncompliance because those are words that are well known by many health care professionals; they capture people's attention and help them understand the benefits for them of a collaborative partnership approach.

Response of Nurse Heather Hart, who works in palliative care:

First I would never attempt to convince a colleague. My colleagues see that I am a happy, keen professional, and that I have a real connection with my patients and their families and enjoy my work. That is an outcome of using a collaborative partnership approach in my practice. It would be very easy for me to go to work and "administer" care to patients and get through my day. There is richness to my nursing that comes from the collaborative relationship that I develop with people. This approach may be potentially time consuming, but it is also more effective and more gratifying. I like that I know the people I am nursing. I know their stories and what is important to them. I have the same time constraints and demands as other staff on my unit. I cope with that by looking for the good things. When you find out where people are coming from, their stories and their experiences, you can be more effective in working with them to plan their care rather that wasting a lot of time and energy on something that is not going to be effective.

Some nurses feel intense responsibility for what happens to families, but with a collaborative partnership approach I do not feel that way because ultimately patients are responsible for their own decisions, and health. A collaborative partnership approach relieves me of the pressure of being the "expert" and "fixer."

Collaborative partnership can enhance your relationships with people. Collaborative partnership can also enrich and give meaning to your nursing practice. It can make nursing rich and exciting. The nurse becomes part of people's stories.

CONCLUSION

The challenges we have addressed in this chapter have highlighted that collaborative partnership does indeed require a delicate balance. This chapter has dealt with some of the special issues, challenges, and circumstances that the nurse has to be aware of to maintain the balance of power in the collaborative partnership relationship. Similar to any relationship, within the collaborative partnership there are expectations for how each partner should conduct themselves and how much they should share in different situations. Collaborative partnership requires a delicate balance between the expert knowledge of the nurse and the expert knowledge of the person, the nurse as professional partner and the nurse as friend, the wishes and desires of the person and their personal safety and that of others, and the nurse giving and the nurse conserving and replenishing energy.

Collaborative partnership is a rewarding approach to nursing practice because it honors and values the person's need for self-determination and personal control and direction. Collaborative partnership reflects a deep valuing and a profound respect for people and their capacity to change, grow, learn, and develop. Not only does the person benefit from collaboration, so does the nurse. In a collaborative relationship, the person learns from the nurse and the nurse learns from the person. As a result, both the nurse and person develop new insights, skills, and a deeper understanding of each other, themselves, the nature of their relationship, and the situation. The insights acquired by both the person and the nurse can enhance their understanding of and ability to deal with other situations and other relationships.

SUGGESTED READING

McCann, T. V., & Baker, H. (2001). Mutual relating: Developing interpersonal relationships in the community. *Journal of Advanced Nursing, 34,* 530-537. This study describes patient and community health nurses' ideas about self-disclosure.

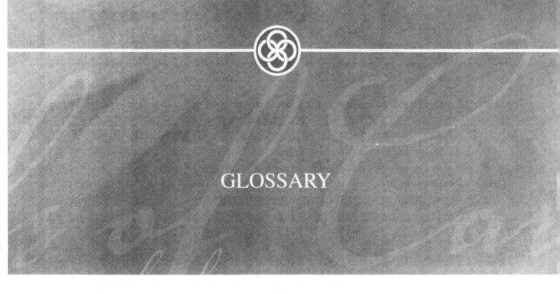

GLOSSARY

ambiguity *(Chapter 2)* the lack of predictability in a collaborative partnership due to the fact that decisions are made by two people rather than just the nurse; collaborative work requires that both the nurse and person be able to tolerate uncertainty and ambiguity for a period of time.

assessment *(Chapter 6)* an ongoing process of systematic reflection on the nature of the nurse-person relationship in order to determine that collaboration is actually occurring; takes place over the course of the relationship, before, during, and after encounters.

attunement skills *(Chapter 4)* a subset of interpersonal skills critical to the collaborative nurse-person relationship; these skills include the ability to read another person's verbal and nonverbal behaviours accurately, and to assess how to pace the work depending on what the person can handle.

collaborative partnership *(Chapter 1)* a type of nurse-person relationship that emphasizes the pursuit of mutually agreed-on, person-centred goals through a dynamic process that requires the active participation and agreement of all partners.

Collaborative Partnership Factors Assessment Guide *(Chapter 4)* originally developed by Dalton (2001) and elaborated on by Gottlieb and Feeley in this book outlines the factors that influence the degree to which the nurse will be able to implement a collaborative partnership approach with the person and the degree to which the person will partner with the nurse; encompasses four major categories of factors: nurse factors; person factors; relationship factors; and environmental, organizational, and situational factors.

constructivism *(Chapter 7)* the theory that people build their own perceptions of how the world operates, selecting from and attending to from the information they observe and hear.

cooperation *(Chapter 1)* a prerequisite for a collaborative partnership; planning and working together in a helpful way (Baggs & Schmitt, 1988).

cultural awareness *(Chapter 7)* the second level of Bushy's (1999) continuum of four levels of cultural-linguistic competence; at this level the professional has an appreciation of and sensitivity to the beliefs, values, and practices of the other person.

cultural knowledge *(Chapter 7)* the third level of Bushy's (1999) continuum of four levels of cultural-linguistic competence; at this level of competence the professional has knowledge of other cultures and uses this in providing care.

enculturation *(Chapter 7)* the fourth level of Bushy's (1999) continuum of four levels of cultural-linguistic competence; at this level the professional develops culturally sensitive care in collaboration with the person, and the person is a partner in planning care.

engagement skills *(Chapter 4)* in a collaborative partnership, the ability of the partners to be involved with the other for the purpose of establishing and maintaining a relationship.

ethnocentrism *(Chapter 7)* the first level of Bushy's (1999) continuum of four levels of cultural-linguistic competence; refers to a lack of cultural sensitivity on the part of the professional, who perceives his or her own cultural affiliation as the standard by which to judge all other cultures.

exploring phase *(Chapter 3)* the first phase of the Spiralling Model of Collaborative Partnership, characterized by activities that enable each partner to get acquainted with the other by exchanging information, establishing trust, and revealing concerns.

fit *(Chapter 4)* the compatibility between the capacities and characteristics of the person and the demands and expectations of the other partner.

indicators *(Chapter 6)* for the purposes of this text, the various signs that suggest the nurse and person are working together collaboratively, including indicators that power is being shared, that there is openness and respect in the relationship, that ambiguity is being tolerated, that reflection is taking place, and that self-awareness is present.

learning style *(Chapter 4)* the way in which a particular individual best acquires an understanding of how something operates in the world, for example, by observing, reading and researching, listening, trial and error, or demonstration.

negotiation *(Chapter 3)* a process of constructive compromising between two partners for the purpose of jointly deciding on priorities in a manner that derives optimum satisfaction for both partners; involves an understanding of the other partner's perspective, the awareness and clear communication of one's own perspective, knowing how to find common ground, and knowing whose perspective should be given greater weight at any given time.

nonjudgmental *(Chapter 2)* showing tolerance and understanding for another person's beliefs, values, behaviours, or perspectives; on the part of the nurse, not criticizing or condemning the person or the person's behaviour even if it departs from the nurse's own values.

openness *(Chapter 2)* within the collaborative partnership, a willingness to develop a relationship with the other person; to share information, ideas, and perspectives with the other person, and to hear what the other has to say; a willingness to experiment, change, or learn something new.

participation *(Chapter 1)* the involvement of the person at some level in the decision-making process or the delivery of a service. Person participation or involvement can be viewed on a continuum that progresses from the passive person and the active health professional to a stage where the person is active and the health professional is inactive.

person *(Chapter 1)* formerly referred to as *patient* or *client,* the nurse's partner in the collaborative partnership, either an individual, a family, a community, or another aggregate group or population. The word *person* carries fewer negative connotations than the other alternatives.

philosophical stance *(Chapter 1)* with respect to collaborative partnership, the combination of the nurse's beliefs, values, and attitudes, oriented towards a collaborative partnership approach, that forms an underlying perspective permeating every interaction and encounter that takes place between the nurse and person, especially relating to their respective roles, how power is shared, how decisions are made, and how care is planned.

power sharing *(Chapter 2)* a mode of interacting in which both the nurse and the person together set their agenda, determine a plan of action that best fits the person's realities, and share the work of implementing the plan; although both partners participate in evaluating the outcomes, it is ultimately the person who decides whether the plan is working.

power-sharing strategies *(Chapter 5)* specific strategies enabling the nurse to approach the person in a manner that will facilitate collaboration; strategies include using language that conveys the idea of partnership, explaining the concept of the collaborative partnership and its benefits, eliciting the person's opinions, inviting the person to share in the flow of information, and determining together the overall framework for the relationship.

readiness *(Chapter 4)* in a collaborative partnership, refers to a willingness to engage in health work or make a change, as well as the intention to act, and a willingness to enter into a relationship with the other partner.

reflection *(Chapter 2)* in a collaborative partnership, an introspective activity involving a continuous internal review and monitoring of the nurse-person encounters, engaged in to help gain self-awareness and awareness of the other person, the dynamics of the relationship, and the impact the behaviour of each person is having on the other.

respect *(Chapter 2)* critical to the success of a collaborative partnership, refers to respect for each partner's roles and responsibilities; seeing the other person as a competent, capable partner who can, to varying degrees and in different ways, participate in the partnership.

reviewing phase *(Chapter 3)* the fourth phase of the Spiralling Model of Collaborative Partnership; involves systematically examining how well the plan worked for the person; enables the person to understand what helped them to achieve their goals.

sharing information *(Chapter 5)* in a collaborative partnership, in contrast to a traditional hierarchical relationship, this refers to the two-way flow of information between nurse and person; a means of sharing power, achieved by allowing the person to ask questions and by providing information to the person.

social climate *(Chapter 4)* the organizational culture in which care is provided, including the values, philosophy, policies, and staffing realities and workload of the health care setting.

Spiralling Model of Collaborative Partnership *(Chapter 3)* the model developed by Moudarres and Ezer (1995) identifying the phases (exploring, zeroing in, working out, reviewing) and processes involved in establishing a collaborative partnership.

traditional hierarchical relationship *(Chapter 1)* traditionally, the dominant form of nurse-person relationship, based on a paternalistic system of values in which the professional assumes the authority and power to make decisions for the person and assumes responsibility for the person's health, and in which the role of the person, in exchange for being taken care of, is to comply with the professional's plan.

working-out phase *(Chapter 3)* the third or problem-solving phase of the Spiralling Model of Collaborative Partnership, involving considering alternative ways of achieving goals and trying out.

zeroing-in phase *(Chapter 3)* the second phase of the Spiralling Model of Collaborative Partnership, characterized by efforts to identify, clarify, and prioritize specific, workable goals.

REFERENCES

PREFACE

Allen, M. (1977). Comparative theories of the expanded role in nursing and its implications for nursing practice: A working paper. *Nursing Papers, 9,* 38-45.

Cameron, G. (2004). Transformational leadership for a health promotion practice. In L. E. Young & V. E. Hayes (Eds.), *Transforming health promotion practice: Concepts, issues and applications* (pp. 99-109). Philadelphia: FA Davis.

Gottlieb, L. N., & Ezer, H. (1997). *A perspective on health, family, learning, and collaborative nursing: A collection of writings on the McGill Model of Nursing.* Montreal: McGill University School of Nursing.

Hartrick, G. (2004). Beyond interpersonal communication: The significance of relationship in health promoting practice. In L. E. Young & V. E. Hayes (Eds.), *Transforming health promotion practice: Concepts, issues and applications* (pp. 49-58). Philadelphia: FA Davis.

CHAPTER 1

Allen, D. (2000). Negotiating the role of expert carers on an adult hospital ward. *Sociology of Health and Illness, 22,* 149-171.

Allen, M. (1977). Comparative theories of the expanded role in nursing and its implications for nursing practice: A working paper. *Nursing Papers, 9,* 38-45.

Attridge, C. B., Budgen, C., Hilton, A., McDavid, J., Molzahn, A., & Purkis, M. E. (1996). *Report of the evaluation of the Comox Valley Nursing Centre.* Victoria, BC: University of Victoria School of Nursing.

Baggs, J. G., & Schmitt, M. H. (1988). Collaboration between nurses and physicians. Image: *Journal of Nursing Scholarship, 20,* 145-149.

Biley, F. (1992). Some determinants that effect patient participation in decision making about nursing care. *Journal of Advanced Nursing, 17,* 414-421.

Brearley, S. (1990). *Patient participation: The literature.* London: Scutari Press.

Brink, P. (1992). Autonomy versus do no harm. *Western Journal of Nursing Research, 14,* 264-266.

Cahill, J. (1996). Patient participation: A concept analysis. *Journal of Advanced Nursing, 24,* 561-571.

Cahill, J. (1998). Patient participation—A review of the literature. *Journal of Clinical Nursing, 7,* 119-128.

Canadian Nurses Association. (1997). *Code of Ethics for Registered Nurses.* Ottawa: Author.

Carey, R. (1989). How values affect the mutual goal setting process with multi-problem families. *Journal of Community Health Nursing, 6,* 7-14.

Carper, B. (1978). Fundamental patterns of knowing in nursing. *Advances in Nursing Science, 1,* 13-23.

Chausse, I. (2003). *Patients' perceptions of collaboration in an outpatient psychiatric setting.* Montreal: McGill University School of Nursing.

Clarke, H. F., & Mass, H. (1998). Comox Valley Nursing Centre: From collaboration to empowerment. *Public Health Nursing, 15,* 216-224.

Coulter, A. (1999). Paternalism or partnership? Patients have grown-up and there's no going back. *British Medical Journal, 319,* 719-720.

Courtney, R., Ballard, E., Fauver, S., Gariota, M., & Holland, L. (1996). The partnership model: Working with individuals, families, and communities toward a new vision of health. *Public Health Nursing, 13,* 177-186.

De Ridder, D. D., Depla, M., Severens, P., & Malsch, M. (1997). Beliefs on coping with illness: A consumer's perspective. *Social Science of Medicine, 44,* 553-559.

DeChillo, N., Koren, P. E., & Schultze, K. H. (1994). From paternalism to partnership: Family and professional collaboration in children's mental health. *American Journal of Orthopsychiatry, 64,* 564-576.

Dennis, K. E. (1990). Patients' control and the information imperative: Clarification and confirmation. *Nursing Research, 39,* 162-166.

Eisenthal, S., & Lazare, A. (1976). Evaluation of the initial interview in a walk-in clinic: The patient's perspective on a "customer approach." *The Journal of Nervous and Mental Disease, 162,* 169-176.

Estabrooks, C. (1998). Will evidence-based nursing practice make practice perfect? *Canadian Journal of Nursing Research, 30,* 15-30.

Ezer, H., Bray, C., & Gros, C. P. (1997). Families' description of the nursing intervention in a randomized control trial. In L. N. Gottlieb & H. Ezer (Eds.), *A perspective on health, family, learning, and collaborative nursing: A collection of writings on the McGill Model of Nursing* (pp. 371-376). Montreal: McGill University School of Nursing.

Gallant, M. H., Beaulieu, M. C., & Carnevale, F. A. (2002). Partnership: An analysis of the concept within the nurse-client relationship. *Journal of Advanced Nursing, 40,* 149-157.

Gottlieb, L. N. (1997). Health promoters: Two contrasting styles in community nursing. In L. N. Gottlieb & H. Ezer (Eds.), *A perspective on health, family, learning, and collaborative nursing: A collection of writings on the McGill Model of Nursing* (pp. 98-109). Montreal: McGill University School of Nursing.

Gottlieb, L. N., & Rowat, K. (1987). The McGill Model of Nursing: A practice-derived model. *Advances in Nursing Science, 9*(4), 51-61. Montreal: McGill University School of Nursing.

Greenfield, S., Kaplan, S., & Ware, J. E. (1985). Expanding patient involvement in care: Effects on patient outcomes. *Annals of Internal Medicine, 102,* 520-528.

Greenfield, S., Kaplan, S. H., Ware, J. E., Martin Yano, E., & Frank, H. L. J. (1988). Patients' participation in medical care: Effects on blood sugar control and quality of life in diabetes. *Journal of General Internal Medicine, 3,* 448-457.

Hall, B. A., & Allan, J. D. (1994). Self in relation: A prolegomenon for holistic nursing. *Nursing Outlook, 42,* 110-116.

Hall, J. A., Roter, D. L., & Katz, N. R. (1988). Meta-analysis of correlates of provider behavior in medical encounters. *Medical Care, 26,* 657-675.

Halstead, R. W., Wagner, L. D., Margo, V., & Ferkol, W. (2002). Counselors' conceptualizations of caring in the counseling relationship. *Counseling and Values, 47,* 34-42.

Hollman, H., & Lorig, K. (2000). Patients as partners in managing chronic disease. *British Medical Journal, 320,* 527-528.

James, T., & Lorentzon, M. (2004). Gathering dust on library shelves or supporting practice?—The fate of research reports in nursing: Examining the literature on evidence-based practice in nursing. In P. Smith, T. James, M. Lorentzon, & R. Pope (Eds.), *Shaping the facts: Evidence-based nursing and health care* (pp. 17-36). Edinburgh: Churchill Livingstone.

Jewell, S. E. (1994). Patient participation: What does it mean to nurses? *Journal of Advanced Nursing, 19,* 433-438.

Kasch, C. (1986). Establishing a collaborative nurse-patient relationship: A distinct focus of nursing action in primary care. *Image: Journal of Nursing Scholarship, 18*(2), 44-47.

Kim, H. S. (1983). Collaborative decision making in nursing practice: A theoretical framework. In P. L. Chinn (Ed.), *Advances in nursing theory development* (pp. 271-283). Rockville, MD: Aspen Systems Corporation.

Kirk, S. (2001). Negotiating lay and professional roles in the care of children with complex health care needs. *Journal of Advanced Nursing, 34,* 593-602.

Kirk, S., & Glendinning, C. (1998). Trends in community care and patient participation: Implications for the roles of informal carers and community nurses in the United Kingdom. *Journal of Advanced Nursing, 28,* 370-381.

Kirschbaum, M. S., & Knafl, K. A. (1996). Major themes in parent-provider relationships: A comparison of life-threatening and chronic illness experiences. *Journal of Family Nursing, 2,* 195-216.

Krouse, H. J., & Roberts, S. J. (1989). Nurse-patient interactive styles: Power, control, and satisfaction. *Western Journal of Nursing Research, 11,* 717-725.

Lenrow, P. B., & Burch, R. W. (1981). Mutual aid and professional services: Opposing or complementary? In B. Gottlieb (Ed.), *Social networks and social supports* (pp. 233-257). Beverly Hills: Sage.

Loiselle, C. G., & Dubois, S. (2003). Getting wired for interactive health communication. *Canadian Nurse, 99,* 22-26.

Lowenberg, J. S. (1989). *Caring & responsibility: The crossroads between holistic practice and traditional medicine.* Philadelphia: University of Pennsylvania Press.

MacIntosh, J., & McCormack, D. (2001). Partnerships identified within primary health care literature. *International Journal of Nursing Studies, 38,* 547-555.

Mayeroff, M. (1972). *On caring.* New York: Harper & Row.

McQueen, A. (2000). Nurse-patient relationships and partnership in hospital care. *Journal of Clinical Nursing, 9,* 723-731.

Moudarres, D., Fabijan, L., & Ezer, H. (2000). *Collaboration: A process and outcomes of mental health nursing.* A paper presented at the annual meeting of the Canadian Federation of Mental Health Nurses, Saskatoon, SK.

MulHall, A. (1998). Nursing, research, and the evidence. *Evidence Based Nursing, 1,* 4-6.

Orlando, I. J. (1961). *The dynamic nurse-patient relationship: Function, process and principles.* New York: GP Putnams's Sons.

Paavilainen, E., & Astedt-Kurki, P. (1997). The client-nurse relationship as experienced by public health nurses: Toward better collaboration. *Public Health Nursing, 14,* 137-142.

Patterson, B. (2001). Myths of empowerment in chronic illness. *Journal of Advanced Nursing, 34,* 574-581.

Patterson, J. M. (1995). Promoting resilience in families experiencing stress. *Pediatric Clinics of North America, 42,* 47-63.

Peplau, H. (1952). *Interpersonal relations in nursing: A conceptual frame of reference for psychodynamic nursing.* New York: Putnam.

Pless, I. B., Feeley, N., Gottlieb, L. N., Rowat, K., Dougherty, G., & Willard, B. (1994). A randomized trial of a nursing intervention to promote the adjustment of children with chronic physical disorders. *Pediatrics, 94,* 70-75.

Pratto, F., & Walker, A. (2001). Dominance in disguise: Power, beneficence and exploitation in personal relationships. In A. Y. Lee-Chai & J. A. Bargh (Eds.),

The use and abuse of power: Multiple perspectives in the causes of corruption. Philadelphia, PA: Psychology Press.

Roberts, K. (2002). Exploring participation: Older people on discharge from hospital. *Journal of Advanced Nursing, 40,* 413-420.

Roberts, S. J., & Krouse, H. J. (1988). Enhancing self-care through active negotiation. *Nurse Practitioner, 13,* 44-52.

Robinson, C. A. (1996). Health care relationships revisited. *Journal of Family Nursing, 2,* 152-173.

Robinson, C. A., & Thorne, S. A. (1984). Strengthening family "interference." *Journal of Advanced Nursing, 9,* 597-602.

Smith, P. (2004). Gathering evidence: The new production of knowledge. In P. Smith, T. James, M. Lorentzon, & R. Pope (Eds.), *Shaping the facts: Evidence-based nursing and health care* (pp. 111-138). Edinburgh: Churchill Livingstone.

Stewart, M. J. (1990). From provider to partner: A conceptual framework for nursing education based on primary health care premises. *Advances in Nursing Science, 12,* 9-27.

Strickland, W. J., & Strickland, D. L. (1996). Partnership building with special populations. *Family Community Health, 19,* 21-34.

Strull, W. M., Lo, B., & Charles, G. (1984). Do patients want to participate in medical decision making? *Journal of the American Medical Association, 252,* 2990-2994.

Suhonen, R. A., Valimaki, M., & Katajisto, J. (2000). Individualized care in a Finnish healthcare organization. *Journal of Clinical Nursing, 9,* 218-227.

Sullivan, T. J. (1998). Consumers in health care Part II: Expert viewpoints. In T. J. Sullivan (Ed.), *Collaboration: A health care imperative* (pp. 561-590). New York: McGraw-Hill.

Thompson, S. C., Pitts, J. S., & Schwankovsky, L. (1993). Preferences for involvement in medical decision-making: Situational and demographic influences. *Patient Education and Counseling, 22,* 133-140.

Thorne, S. E., & Robinson, C. A. (1988). Reciprocal trust in health care relationships. *Journal of Advanced Nursing, 13,* 782-789.

Trnobranski, P. H. (1994). Nurse-patient negotiation: Assumption or reality? *Journal of Advanced Nursing, 19,* 733-737.

Waterworth, S., & Luker, K. A. (1990). Reluctant collaborators: Do patients want to be involved in decisions concerning care? *Journal of Advanced Nursing, 15,* 971-976.

Westberg, J., & Jason, H. (1996). Fostering healthy behavior. In S. H. Woolf, S. Jonas, & R. Lawrence (Eds.), *Health promotion and disease prevention in clinical practice* (pp. 145-162). Baltimore: Williams & Wilkins.

Williamson, J. A. (1981). Mutual interaction: A model of nursing practice. *Nursing Outlook, 29,* 104-107.

Young, L. E., & Hayes, V. E. (2002). *Transforming health promotion practice: Concepts, issues and applications.* Philadelphia: FA Davis.

CHAPTER 2

Allen, D. (2000). Negotiating the role of expert carers on an adult hospital ward. *Sociology of Health and Illness, 22,* 149-171.

Allen, M. (1977). Comparative theories of the expanded role in nursing and its implications for nursing practice: A working paper. *Nursing Papers, 9,* 38-45.

Attridge, C. B., Budgen, C., Hilton, A., McDavid, J., Molzahn, A., & Purkis, M. E. (1996). *Report of the evaluation of the Comox Valley Nursing Centre.* Victoria, BC: University of Victoria School of Nursing.

Banks, S., Crossman, D., Poel, J., & Stewart, M. (1997). Partnerships among health professionals and self-help group members. *Canadian Journal of Occupational Therapy, 64,* 259-269.

Bidmead, C., Davis, H., & Day, C. (2002). Partnership working: What does it really mean? *Community Practitioner, 75,* 256-259.

Clarke, B., James, C., & Kelly, J. (1996). Reflective practice: Reviewing the issues and refocusing the debate. *International Journal of Nursing Studies, 33,* 171-180.

Clarke, H. F., & Mass, H. (1998). Comox Valley Nursing Centre: From collaboration to empowerment. *Public Health Nursing, 15,* 216-224.

Coulter, A. (1999). Paternalism or partnership? Patients have grown up and there's no going back. *British Medical Journal, 319,* 719-720.

Courtney, R., Ballard, E., Fauver, S., Gariota, M., & Holland, L. (1996). The partnership model: Working with individuals, families, and communities toward a new vision of health. *Public Health Nursing, 13,* 177-186.

Greenwood, J. (1998). The role of reflection in single and double loop learning. *Journal of Advanced Nursing, 27,* 1048-1053.

Henderson, S. (2003). Power imbalance between nurses and patients: A potential inhibitor of partnership in care. *Journal of Clinical Nursing, 12,* 501-508.

Henneman, E. A., Lee, J. L., & Cohen, J. I. (1995). Collaboration: A concept analysis. *Journal of Advanced Nursing, 21,* 103-109.

Jansson, A., Petersson, K., & Uden, G. (2001). Nurses' first encounters with parents of newborn children—Public health nurses' views of a good meeting. *Journal of Clinical Nursing, 10,* 140-151.

Kirschbaum, M. S., & Knafl, K. A. (1996). Major themes in parent-provider relationships: A comparison of life-threatening and chronic illness experiences. *Journal of Family Nursing, 2,* 195-216.

Lahdenpera, T. S., & Kyngas, H. A. (2001). Levels of compliance shown by hypertensive patients and their attitude toward their illness. *Journal of Advanced Nursing, 34,* 189-195.

MacGillivary, H., & Nelson, G. (1998). Partnership in mental health: What it is and how to do it. *Canadian Journal of Rehabilitation, 12,* 71-83.

MacIntosh, J., & McCormack, D. (2001). Partnerships identified within primary health care literature. *International Journal of Nursing Studies, 38,* 547-555.

McCann, T. V., & Baker, H. (2001). Mutual relating: Developing interpersonal relationships in the community. *Journal of Advanced Nursing, 34,* 530-537.

McQueen, A. (2000). Nurse-patient relationships and partnership in hospital care. *Journal of Clinical Nursing, 9,* 723-731.

Nordgren, S., & Fridlund, B. (2001). Patients' perceptions of self-determination as expressed in the context of care. *Journal of Advanced Nursing, 35,* 117-125.

Paavilainen, E., & Astedt-Kurki, P. (1997). The client-nurse relationship as experienced by public health nurses: Toward better collaboration. *Public Health Nursing, 14,* 137-142.

Robinson, C. A. (1996). Health care relationships revisited. *Journal of Family Nursing, 2,* 152-173.

Schon, D. (1987). *The reflective practitioner: How professionals think in action.* New York: Basic Books.

Thorne, S. E., & Robinson, C. A. (1988). Reciprocal trust in health care relationships. *Journal of Advanced Nursing, 13,* 782-789.

CHAPTER 3

Bidmead, C., Davis, H., & Day, C. (2002). Partnership working: What does it really mean? *Community Practitioner, 75,* 256-259.

Courtney, R., Ballard, E., Fauver, S., Gariota, M., & Holland, L. (1996). The partnership model: Working with individuals, families, and communities toward a new vision of health. *Public Health Nursing, 13,* 177-186.

Gottlieb, L. N., & Rowat, K. (1987). The McGill Model of Nursing: A practice-derived model. *Advances in Nursing Science, 9*(4), 51-61.

Jansson, A., Petersson, K., & Uden, G. (2001). Nurses' first encounters with parents of newborn children—Public health nurses' views of a good meeting. *Journal of Clinical Nursing, 10,* 140-151.

Moudarres, D., & Ezer, H. (1995, December). *Collaboration with individuals, families, and groups in the community.* Paper presented at International Conference on Community Health Centres, Montreal.

Moudarres, D., Ezer, H., & Schein, C. (1997). *Collaboration: A process and outcomes of community health nursing.* Paper presented at the Canadian National Home Care Association Conference, Montreal.

Moudarres, D., Fabijan, L., & Ezer, H. (2000). *Collaboration: A process and outcomes of nursing practice.* Paper presented at the Annual Meeting of the Canadian Federation of Mental Health Nurses, Saskatoon, Sask.

Roberts, S. J., & Krouse, H. J. (1988). Enhancing self-care through active nego-tiation. *Nurse Practitioner, 13,* 44-52.

Roberts, S. J., & Krouse, H. J. (1990). Negotiation as a strategy to empowering self-care. *Holistic Nursing Practice, 4,* 30-36.

Williamson, J. A. (1981). Mutual interaction: A model of nursing practice. *Nursing Outlook, 29,* 104-107.

CHAPTER 4

Benner, P., Hooper-Kyriakidis, P., & Stannard, D. (1999). *Clinical wisdom and interventions in critical care: A thinking-in-action approach.* Philadelphia: WB Saunders Company.

Biley, F. (1992). Some determinants that effect patient participation in decision making about nursing care. *Journal of Advanced Nursing, 17,* 414-421.

Bottorff, J., Steele, R., Davis, B., Porterfield, P., Garossino, C., & Shaw, M. (2000). Facilitating day-to-day decision making in palliative care. *Cancer Nursing, 23,* 141-150.

Cahill, J. (1998). Patient participation—A review of the literature. *Journal of Clinical Nursing, 7,* 119-128.

Chan, L. (2003). *Having their say: The challenges of addressing the concerns of adolescents with chronic illness and their families in an ambulatory setting.* Unpublished manuscript, McGill University School of Nursing, Montreal.

Dalton, C. (2001). *Conditions for collaboration framework.* Unpublished manu-script. McGill University School of Nursing, Montreal.

Dalton, C., & Gottlieb, L. N. (2003). The concept of readiness to change. *Journal of Advanced Nursing, 42,* 108-117.

DeChillo, N. (1993). Collaboration between social workers and families of patients with mental illness. *Families in Society: The Journal of Contempo-rary Human Services, 74,* 104-115.

Espezel, H. J. E., & Canam, C. J. (2003). Parent-nurse interactions: Care of hos-pitalized children. *Journal of Advanced Nursing, 44,* 34-41.

Kim, H. S. (1983). Collaborative decision making in nursing practice: A theo-retical framework. In P. L. Chinn (Ed.), *Advances in nursing theory develop-ment* (pp. 271-283). Rockville, MD: Aspen Systems Corporation.

Kirk, S. (2001). Negotiating lay and professional roles in the care of children with complex health care needs. *Journal of Advanced Nursing, 34,* 593-602.

Kirk, S., & Glendinning, C. (1998). Trends in community care and patient par-ticipation: Implications for the roles of informal carers and community nurses in the United Kingdom. *Journal of Advanced Nursing, 28,* 370-381.

Krouse, H. J., & Roberts, S. J. (1989). Nurse-patient interactive styles: Power, control, and satisfaction. *Western Journal of Nursing Research, 11,* 717-725.

Lenrow, P. B., & Burch, R. W. (1981). Mutual aid and professional services: Opposing or complementary? In B. Gottlieb (Ed.), *Social networks and social supports* (pp. 233-257). Beverly Hills: Sage.

McCann, T. V., & Baker, H. (2001). Mutual relating: Developing interpersonal relationships in the community. *Journal of Advanced Nursing, 34,* 530-537.

McKeachie, W. J. (1999). *Teaching tips: Strategies, research and theory for college and university teachers* (10th ed.). Boston: Houghton Mifflin Company.

Murphy, F., Taylor, G., & Townshend, J. (1997). Assessing and promoting families' readiness for change and growth. In L. N. Gottlieb & H. Ezer (Eds.), *A perspective on health, family, learning, and collaborative nursing: A collection of writings on the McGill Model of Nursing* (pp. 365-369). Montreal: McGill University School of Nursing.

Naylor, D. (2003). *National advisory committee on SARS and public health.* Ottawa: Health Canada.

Nordgren, S., & Fridlund, B. (2001). Patients' perceptions of self-determination as expressed in the context of care. *Journal of Advanced Nursing, 35,* 117-125.

Patterson, B. (2001). Myths of empowerment in chronic illness. *Journal of Advanced Nursing, 34,* 574-581.

Sainio, C., Eriksson, E., & Lauri, S. (2001). Patient participation in decision making about care: The cancer patient's point of view. *Cancer Nursing, 24,* 172-179.

CHAPTER 5

Atkins, S., & Murphy, K. (1993). Reflection: A review of the literature. *Journal of Advanced Nursing, 18,* 1188-1192.

Bidmead, C., Davis, H., & Day, C. (2002). Partnership working: What does it really mean? *Community Practitioner, 75,* 256-259.

Bottorff, J., Steele, R., Davis, B., Porterfield, P., Garossino, C., & Shaw, M. (2000). Facilitating day-to-day decision making in palliative care. *Cancer Nursing, 23,* 141-150.

Feeley, N., & Gottlieb, L. N. (2000). Nursing approaches for working with family strengths and resources. *Journal of Family Nursing, 6,* 9-23.

Greenwood, J. (1998). The role of reflection in single and double loop learning. *Journal of Advanced Nursing, 27,* 1048-1053.

Haug, M. R. (1996). Elements in physician/patient interactions in late life. *Research on Aging, 18,* 32-51.

Heath, H. (1998). Keeping a reflective practice diary: A practical guide. *Nurse Education Today, 18,* 592-598.

Henderson, S. (2003). Power imbalance between nurses and patients: A potential inhibitor of partnership in care. *Journal of Clinical Nursing, 12,* 501-508.

Jansson, A., Petersson, K., & Uden, G. (2001). Nurses' first encounters with parents of newborn children—Public health nurses' views of a good meeting. *Journal of Clinical Nursing, 10,* 140-151.

Johns, C. (1994). Nuances of reflection. *Journal of Clinical Nursing, 3,* 71-75.

Kasch, C. (1986). Establishing a collaborative nurse-patient relationship: A distinct focus of nursing action in primary care. *Image: Journal of Nursing Scholarship, 18*(2), 44-47.

Leahey, M., & Harper-Jaques, S. (1996). Family-nurse relationships: Core assumptions and clinical implications. *Journal of Family Nursing, 2,* 133-151.

Lenrow, P. B., & Burch, R. W. (1981). Mutual aid and professional services: Opposing or complementary? In B. Gottlieb (Ed.), *Social networks and social supports* (pp. 233-257). Beverly Hills: Sage.

Mitcheson, J., & Cowley, S. (2003). Empowerment or control? An analysis of the extent to which client participation is enabled during health visitor/client interactions using a structured health needs assessment tool. *International Journal of Nursing Studies, 40,* 413-426.

Patterson, B. (2001). Myths of empowerment in chronic illness. *Journal of Advanced Nursing, 34,* 574-581.

Roberts, K. (2002). Exploring participation: Older people on discharge from hospital. *Journal of Advanced Nursing, 40,* 413-420.

Robinson, C. A. (1996). Health care relationships revisited. *Journal of Family Nursing, 2,* 152-173.

Sainio, C., Eriksson, E., & Lauri, S. (2001). Patient participation in decision making about care: The cancer patient's point of view. *Cancer Nursing, 24,* 172-179.

Tapp, D. (2000). The ethics of relational stance in family nursing: Resisting the view of "nurse as expert." *Journal of Family Nursing, 6,* 69-91.

Thorne, S. E., & Robinson, C. A. (1988). Reciprocal trust in health care relationships. *Journal of Advanced Nursing, 13,* 782-789.

Walker, E., & Dewar, B. J. (2001). How do we facilitate carers' involvement in decision making? *Journal of Advanced Nursing, 34,* 329-337.

CHAPTER 6

Allen, M. (1977). Comparative theories of the expanded role in nursing and its implications for nursing practice: A working paper. *Nursing Papers, 9,* 38-45.

Greenwood, J. (1998). The role of reflection in single and double loop learning. *Journal of Advanced Nursing, 27,* 1048-1053.

Karhila, P., Kettunen, T., Poskiparta, M., & Liimatainen, L. (2003). Negotiation in type 2 diabetes counseling: From problem recognition to mutual acceptance during lifestyle counseling. *Qualitative Health Research, 13,* 1205-1224.

Lahdenpera, T. S., & Kyngas, H. A. (2001). *Journal of Advanced Nursing, 34,* 189-195.

Walker, E., & Dewar, B. J. (2001). How do we facilitate carers' involvement in decision making? *Journal of Advanced Nursing, 34,* 329-337.

CHAPTER 7

Allen, D. (2000). Negotiating the role of expert carers on an adult hospital ward. *Sociology of Health and Illness, 22,* 149-171.

Bushy, A. (1999). Resiliency and social support. In J. G. Sebastian & A. Bushy (Eds.), *Special populations in the community: Advances in reducing health disparities* (pp. 189-195). Rockville, MD: Aspen Publishers.

Cioffi, J. (2003). Communicating with culturally and linguistically diverse patients in an acute care setting: Nurses' experiences. *International Journal of Nursing Studies, 40,* 299-306.

Egan, G. (2002). *The skilled helper: A problem-management and opportunity-development approach to helping* (7th ed.). Pacific Grove, CA: Brooks/Cole Publisher.

Ekstrom, D. N. (1999). Gender and perceived nurse caring in nurse-patient dyads. *Journal of Advanced Nursing, 29,* 1393-1401.

Friedman, M. M., Bowden, V. R., & Jones, E. G. (2003). The family nursing process. In *Family nursing: Research, theory and practice* (5th ed, pp. 173-211). Upper Saddle River, NJ: Prentice-Hall.

Hall, J. A., & Roter, D. L. (2002). Do patients talk differently to male and female physicians? A meta-analytic review. *Patient Education and Counseling, 48,* 217-224.

Jansson, A., Petersson, K., & Uden, G. (2001). Nurses' first encounters with parents of newborn children—Public health nurses' views of a good meeting. *Journal of Clinical Nursing, 10,* 140-151.

Kirk, S. (2001). Negotiating lay and professional roles in the care of children with complex health care needs. *Journal of Advanced Nursing, 34,* 593-602.

Kulbok, P. A., Gates, M. F., Vincenzi, A. E., & Schultz, P. R. (1999). Focus on community: Directions for nursing knowledge development. *Journal of Advanced Nursing, 29,* 1188-1196.

Lynch, E. W. (1998). Developing cross-cultural competence. In E. W. Lynch & M. J. Hanson (Eds.), *Developing cross-cultural competence: A guide for working with children and their families* (pp. 47-85). Baltimore: Paul H Brookes Publishing.

Mahoney, M. (1991). Constructivism and self-organization. In *Human change processes,* 95-117. New York: Basic Books.

Patterson, B. (2001). Myths of empowerment in chronic illness. *Journal of Advanced Nursing, 34,* 574-581.

Pender, N. J., Murdaugh, C. L., & Parsons, M. A. (2002). Health promotion in vulnerable populations. In N. J. Pender, *Health promotion in nursing practice* (4th ed, pp. 103-114). Upper Saddle River, NJ: Prentice Hall.

Ransom, D. C., Fisher, L., Phillips, S., Kokes, R. F., & Weiss, R. (1990). The logic of measurement in family research. In T. W. Draper & A. C. Marcos (Eds.), *Family variables: Conceptualization, measurement and use* (pp. 48-63). Newbury Park, CA: Sage Publications.

Reimer Kirkham, S. (1998). Nurses' descriptions of caring for culturally diverse clients. *Clinical Nursing Research, 7,* 125-147.

Roberts, K. (2002). Exploring participation: Older people on discharge from hospital. *Journal of Advanced Nursing, 40,* 413-420.

Sainio, C., & Lauri, S. (2003). Cancer patients' decision-making regarding treatment and nursing care. *Journal of Advanced Nursing, 41,* 250-260.

Siegel, D. J. (1999). Representations: Modes of processing and the construction of reality. In *The developing mind: Toward a neurobiology of interpersonal experience* (pp. 160-205). New York: The Guilford Press.

Steen, S., & Schwartz, P. (1995). Communication, gender and power: Homosexual couples as a case study. In M. A. Fitzpatrick & A. L. Vangelisti (Eds.), *Explaining family interactions* (pp. 310-343). Thousand Oaks, CA: Sage Publications.

Street, R. L. (2002). Gender differences in health care provider-patient communication: Are they due to style, stereotypes, or accommodation? *Patient Education and Counseling, 48,* 201-206.

Styles, M. (1996). Conceptualizations of advanced nursing practice. In A. Hamric, J. Sprouse & C. Hansen (Eds.), *Advanced nursing practice: An integrated approach* (pp. 25-41). Toronto: WB Saunders.

Tannen, D. (1990). *You just don't understand.* New York: Ballantine Books.

Thompson, S. C., Pitts, J. S., & Schwankovsky, L. (1993). Preferences for involvement in medical decision-making: Situational and demographic influences. *Patient Education and Counseling, 22,* 133-140.

van den Brink-Muinen, A., van Dulmen, S., Messerli-Rohrbach, & Bensing, J. (2002). Do gender-dyads have different communication patterns? A comparative study in Western-European general practices. *Patient Education and Counseling, 48,* 253-264.

CHAPTER 8

Allen, D. (2000). Negotiating the role of expert carers on an adult hospital ward. *Sociology of Health and Illness, 22,* 149-171.

Benner, P., & Wrubel, J. (1989). *The primacy of caring.* New York: Addison-Wesley.

Browne, G., Roberts, J., Byrne, C., Gafni, A., Weir, R., & Majundar, B. (2001). The costs and effects of addressing the needs of vulnerable populations: Results of 10 years of research. *Canadian Journal of Nursing Research, 33,* 65-76.

Cahill, J. (1998). Patient participation—A review of the literature. *Journal of Clinical Nursing, 7,* 119-128.

Carper, B. (1978). Fundamental patterns of knowing in nursing. *Advances in Nursing Science, 1,* 13-23.

Chinn, P. L., & Kramer, M. K. (2004). *Integrated knowledge development in nursing* (6th ed.). St. Louis, MO: Mosby.

Feeley, N., & Gerez-Lirette, T. (1992). Development of professional practice based on the McGill Model of Nursing in an ambulatory care setting. *Journal of Advanced Nursing, 17,* 801-808.

Henderson, S. (2002). Influences on patient participations and decision-making in care. *Professional Nurse, 17,* 521-525.

McBride, C. M., & Rimer, B. K. (1999). Using the telephone to improve health behaviour and health service delivery. *Patient Education and Counseling, 37,* 3-18.

McCann, T. V., & Baker, H. (2001). Mutual relating: Developing interpersonal relationships in the community. *Journal of Advanced Nursing, 34,* 530-537.

Murphy, F. (1994). A staff development program to support the incorporation of the McGill Model of Nursing into an out-patient clinic department. *Journal of Advanced Nursing, 20,* 750-754.

Roberts, K. (2002). Exploring participation: Older people on discharge from hospital. *Journal of Advanced Nursing, 40,* 413-420.

Sainio, C., & Lauri, S. (2003). Cancer patients' decision-making regarding treatment and nursing care. *Journal of Advanced Nursing, 41,* 250-260.

Thompson, S. C., Pitts, J. S., & Schwankovsky, L. (1993). Preferences for involvement in medical decision-making: Situational and demographic influences. *Patient Education and Counseling, 22,* 133-140.

Thorne, S. E., Nyhlin, K. T., & Paterson, B. L. (2000). Attitudes toward patient expertise in chronic illness. *International Journal of Nursing Studies, 37,* 303-311.

Walsh, K. (1997). Encounters, endings and temporality in psychiatric nursing. *Journal of Advanced Nursing, 25,* 485-491.

GLOSSARY

Baggs, J. G., & Schmitt, M. H. (1988). Collaboration between nurses and physicians. Image: *Journal of Nursing Scholarship, 20,* 145-149.

Bushy, A. (1999). Resiliency and social support. In J. G. Sebastian & A. Bushy (Eds.), *Special populations in the community: Advances in reducing health disparities* (pp. 189-195). Rockville, MD: Aspen Publishers.

Dalton, C. (2001). *Conditions for collaboration framework.* Unpublished manuscript. McGill University School of Nursing, Montreal.

Moudarres, D., & Ezer, H. (1995, December). *Collaboration with individuals, families, and groups in the community.* Paper presented at International Conference in Community Health Centres, Montreal.

INDEX

Note: Page numbers followed by *f* indicate figures; *t*, tables; *b*, boxes.

COLLABORATIVE PARTNERSHIP FACTS

FACT ▶ In any partnership, one partner may assume more responsibility or play a more active role at any given time, and then responsibility may shift to the other partner at other points in time. The collaborative nature of a relationship often shifts over the course of one encounter or over the course of a relationship (page 30).

FACT ▶ The knowledge and experience of both the nurse and the person are essential for effective care. The nurse has expert knowledge and uses this in the collaborative partnership. The nurse and the person share responsibility for what happens (page 29).

FACT ▶ People are more likely to commit to a plan of action if they have played a role in designing the plan or treatment regimen or in customizing the plan to meet their needs and particular situation (page 94).

FACT ▶ Asking the person about his or her perspective on the situation and taking this perspective into consideration when devising the plan of care is only a first step in the process of working collaboratively, but it is not true collaborative partnership. The person has to be a partner in decision making, not just a consultant (page 46).

FACT ▶ All people have goals, because humans are by nature goal directed. However, some people have difficulty either identifying or describing to others what they want to achieve (page 48).

FACT ▶ The nurse's professional knowledge and expertise are important in a collaborative partnership relationship. The person has his or her own goals, and the nurse too may have goals for the person. A collaborative partnership is effective in part because the knowledge, expertise, and contributions of both partners are valued and tapped (page 29).

FACT ▶ In a collaborative relationship the person learns from the nurse and the nurse learns from the person. As a result, both the nurse and the person develop new insights, skills, and a deeper understanding of each other, themselves, the nature of the relationship, and the situation (page 150).

FACT ▶ Partnerships work best when there is a clear understanding of one's own role and the role of the other. When each partner has a clear understanding of his or her own role and what to expect from the other partner, then the stage is set for a well-functioning partnership (page 44).

FACT ▶ Collaboration involves the nurse recognizing, getting in tune with, and working with each person's unique capacities and competencies. Collaborative partnership is possible with the majority of people regardless of their level of education or ability to articulate their needs and define their goals (page 122).

FACT ▶ The collaborative partnership relationship often leads people to feel secure because they have come to trust in themselves and the nurse. Those feelings of security may help the person to tap into his or her own strengths and draw on resources to meet life's challenges (page 148).

FACT ▶ Nurses often meet people during periods of change, crisis, and life transition, and during these times, people are usually more vulnerable and more open to forming relationships with nurses. This can certainly expedite the development of a collaborative partnership (page 126).